PUBLIC LAW AND HEALTH SERVICE ACCOUNTABILITY

STATE OF HEALTH SERIES

Edited by Chris Ham, Director of the Health Services
Management Centre, University of Birmingham

Current and forthcoming titles

Financing Health Care in the 1990s
John Appleby

Patients, Policies and Politics
John Butler

Public Law and Health Service Accountability
Diane Longley

Hospitals in Transition
Tim Packwood, Justin Keen and Martin Buxton

Planned Markets and Public Competition
Richard B. Saltman and Casten von Otter

*Whose Standards? Consumer and Professional Standards in
Health Care*
Charlotte Williamson

PUBLIC LAW AND HEALTH SERVICE ACCOUNTABILITY

Diane Longley

Open University Press
Buckingham · Philadelphia

Open University Press
Celtic Court
22 Ballmoor
Buckingham
MK18 1XW

and
1900 Frost Road, Suite 101
Bristol, PA 19007, USA

First Published 1993

A catalogue record of this book is
available from the British Library

Library of Congress Cataloging-in-Publication Data

Longley, Diane, 1945–
    Public law and health service accountability/Diane Longley.
        p.   cm. – (State of health series)
    Includes bibliographical references and index.
    ISBN 0–335–09685–9 (pb)   ISBN 0–335–09686–7 (hb)
    1. National Health Service (Great Britain)   2. Medical policy Great
Britain.   3. Medical care – law and legislation – Great Britain.
I. Title.   II. Series.
    [DNLM: 1. Delivery of Health Care – Great Britain – legislation.
2. Delivery of Health Care – organization & administration – Great
Britain.   3. Health Policy – Great Britain.   4. State Medicine – Great
Britain – legislation.   5. State Medicine – organization &
administration – Great Britain. W 275 FA1 L8p]
RA395.G6L66 1992   362.1′0941 – dc20
DNLM/DLC for Library of Congress   92–13011
                                                                                        CIP

Typeset by Type Study, Scarborough
Printed in Great Britain by St Edmundsbury Press
Bury St Edmunds, Suffolk

To Vicky and Bill Baldwin

CONTENTS

SERIES EDITOR'S INTRODUCTION

Health services in many developed countries have come under critical scrutiny in recent years. In part this is because of increasing expenditure, much of it funded from public sources, and the pressure this has put on governments seeking to control public spending. Also important has been the perception that resources allocated to health services are not always deployed in an optimal fashion. Thus at a time when the scope for increasing expenditure is extremely limited, there is a need to search for ways of using existing budgets more efficiently. A further concern has been the desire to ensure access to health care of various groups on an equitable basis. In some countries this has been linked to a wish to enhance patient choice and to make service providers more responsive to patients as 'consumers'.

Underlying these specific concerns are a number of more fundamental developments which have a significant bearing on the performance of health services. Three are worth highlighting. First, there are demographic changes, including the ageing population and the decline in the proportion of the population of working age. These changes will both increase the demand for health care and at the same time limit the ability of health services to respond to this demand.

Second, advances in medical science will also give rise to new demands within the health services. These advances cover a range of possibilities, including innovations in surgery, drug therapy, screening and diagnosis. The pace of innovation is likely to quicken as the end of the century approaches, with significant implications for the funding and provision of services.

Third, public expectations of health services are rising as those who use services demand higher standards of care. In part, this is stimulated by developments within the health service, including the availability of new technology. More fundamentally, it stems from the emergence of a more educated and informed population, in which people are accustomed to being treated as consumers rather than patients.

Against this background, policy makers in a number of countries are reviewing the future of health services. Those countries which have traditionally relied on a market in health care are making greater use of regulation and planning. Equally, those countries which have traditionally relied on regulation and planning are moving towards a more competitive approach. In no country is there complete satisfaction with existing methods of financing and delivery, and everywhere there is a search for new policy instruments.

The aim of this series is to contribute to debate about the future of health services through an analysis of major issues in health policy. These issues have been chosen because they are both of current interest and of enduring importance. The series is intended to be accessible to students and informed lay readers as well as to specialists working in this field. The aim is to go beyond a textbook approach to health policy analysis and to encourage authors to move debate about their issue forward. In this sense, each book presents a summary of current research and thinking, and an exploration of future policy directions.

Professor Chris Ham
Director of the Health Services Management Centre,
University of Birmingham

PREFACE AND ACKNOWLEDGEMENTS

The National Health Service and Community Care Act received the royal assent on 29 June 1990 giving legislative backing to health service reforms initially proposed in the white paper 'Working for Patients', which heralded the third major reorganization in the National Health Service in recent years.

Prior to the 1974 restructuring, Rudolf Klein had commented that although the NHS was one of the most pervasive of all government services there had been a paucity of academic debate about the problems of trying to reconcile public accountability, managerial efficiency and professional attitudes within the system (1974, p. 364). Almost 20 years on this book seeks partially to fill that vacuum by examining the relationship between the processes of accountability and management within the health service, in the light of the recent Act and changes that are currently in progress.

The arguments put forward rest on a firm belief in a constitutional backcloth for the operation of all public activity and arrangements for governing. By definition public power is exercised on behalf of all citizens. Each and every one of us has a right to be concerned with its application, which includes moral, political and practical matters. The challenge for society and the organization of its institutions is to try to provide a means of drawing together those three inherent elements in such a way as to safeguard the citizen, both as an individual and as a member of society, from arbitrary decision-making. It will be suggested that a possible solution lies in the use of the skills and techniques of law as a means of providing the necessary building fabric with which to frame the legitimate exercise of public power and public management.

Our health care delivery system is in ferment. The rapid and profound changes that are taking place may or may not lead to improvement. In the face of these changes we need to understand the broad context of the role of law in health policy as well as its more concrete detailed expression. We need to know where our health care system has come from, why it is the way it is, where it is going and what its aspirations are and what are the forces influencing and shaping fundamental choices. It is this latter consideration which is the focus of what follows. We need to learn so that we can understand what our expectations for our health care system are, and then work towards a realization or adjustment of those expectations by setting realistic standards for improvement.

The underlying theme throughout this book is that health care is a political issue in its truest sense; a matter of a social entitlement to be moulded and allocated according to explicit social choices and to be protected from becoming a commodity, shaped and distributed by largely unaccountable 'market' tendencies that focus at least rhetorically on individual consumption. Learning and social choice require relevant information; consequently a great deal of emphasis needs to be put on the requirement for openness in management processes and professional activity. It is argued that the introduction of norms of conduct for the management of health services, designed to secure acceptance of policy decisions and promote a better understanding of the reasonableness of decisions and the processes of decision-making, might eventually lead to a more stable and satisfactory organization.

The main focus of the following chapters is public accountability for the allocation of resources. Consequently there is no discussion of any personal accountability of the medical profession to patients for clinical practice on an individual basis. Those issues are covered extensively in other literature and are I feel outside the scope of this text, as they involve private law procedures for the tort of medical negligence. However, a brief comment is made in Chapter 4 on the implications of medical malpractice litigation for health authority budgets.

On a personal note, I would like to acknowledge the support I have received from all my friends and colleagues at the Centre for Socio-Legal Studies, the University of Sheffield during the writing of this book. My thanks go especially to Norman Lewis for stimulating my interest in public law and giving me the confidence to eventually put 'pen to paper', to Mary Seneviratne for her constant encouragement, to Ian Harden for his many discussions of some of the difficulties of NHS reorganization and to Rand Rosenblatt for the courtesy he showed me on my visit to the USA and the contribution of his extensive knowledge of American health law. My thanks also go to the British Academy and the Economic and Social Research Council who each contributed funding towards the research which in part forms the basis of the book. Last but certainly not least, my gratitude goes to my long-suffering family, who have seen me through so many trials and tribulations this year. In some ways I can liken the effect of writing this book to the effect that contracting is having on District Health Authorities; it has made me think through my priorities. I therefore make no apologies for this my first and in all probability, my last book.

1

DIAGNOSTIC DEFICIENCIES: HEALTH POLICY, PUBLIC LAW AND PUBLIC MANAGEMENT

BACKGROUND

Although the promotion and maintenance of good health has long been recognized to be a fundamental and legitimate public policy objective the actual provision of health care services remains one of the most problematic socio-economic functions of the modern state. Whatever the actual level of government involvement in the delivery and funding of services the provision of health care has been a dominant topic in the majority of health care systems over the last four or five decades. Frequently amongst the most urgent and traumatic issues confronted are those of priority setting and resource allocation. In the UK the difficulties have become steadily more visible and acute, arousing extensive debate and concern about the future organization of health care provision and the viability of the National Health Service (NHS).

The declared aims of the NHS at its inception were exemplary; they were to promote better health, to ensure equal access to care and to provide comprehensive coverage, free at the point of entry. Market allocation of resources was rejected and health care was considered to be a matter of social entitlement to be both provided and funded from public resources. By providing an organizational framework for national coordination of the allocation and distribution of resources the NHS was considered to be an expedient and relatively economic solution to the enormous task of delivering health care. Despite the contentious debates prior to the enactment of the National Health Service Act 1946 and initial dissension from the medical profession about some aspects of the new health care provisions, the initial aims of the NHS have commanded and continued to maintain substantial support and respect from all quarters.

In many ways the NHS has proved to be a resounding success. It has major strengths; it is comparatively comprehensive, equitable and accessible and by international comparison it provides relatively good standards of care at low overhead cost. But the sheer scale and diversity of health services required, the continual development of new and highly technical procedures for diagnosis and treatment, not to mention the toll of ever-increasing demand have exerted recurrent pressures on the system which have led to severe problems in sustaining or even attaining primary objectives. As expectations in health care have expanded so has the outlay of cost in terms of labour and equipment. Although in a few areas such as laundering, catering and certain laboratory services the introduction of more advanced mechanization and technology may lower some costs, the scope for reduction of labour in the health service is often less than in many other industries or organizations. Advances in medical knowledge tend to expand productivity and encourage the development of clinical specialities which require highly trained staff and the use of increasingly sophisticated equipment. But at the same time these developments also have a tendency to increase the number of unnecessary and inappropriate services in some areas, which may eventually lead to an inequitable allocation and inefficient use of resources. Not surprisingly such 'medical inflation' has caused government to seek means to control escalating costs and to secure 'value for money' and a more efficient use of resources in the provision of health care as a matter of some urgency.

In addition to the difficulties arising from medical inflation, almost from the outset, there has been a continual problem with the overall planning and co-ordination of the different parts of the service. The NHS has been subject to numerous reports which have highlighted 'a continuing degree of uncertainty about the necessary organisational, administrative and financial consequences of the ideals and aspirations of the service' (Carrier and Kendall, 1990, p. 4). In response, a series of well-documented, pragmatic and incremental changes have occurred which have typically resulted in the strengthening of the NHS management structure and an increasing emphasis on cost containment, with little consideration of the overall implications of these moves. Initial changes were concerned with achieving savings primarily in non-clinical areas of NHS operations. But in more recent years attempts have been made to involve clinicians, who ultimately determine use of resources in the NHS, in taking a share of responsibility for operating within budgetary limits. However, both the purpose and effectiveness of some of these efficiency improving measures is open to question and has given rise to concern that in practice savings would be achieved through cuts in services rather than through any sustained increase in efficiency.

As health care spending has failed to be contained within prescribed cash-limits, health care provision itself has frequently been constrained by means which are not always explicit. Service rationing and hence health policy has therefore come to be more the result of tacit action rather than open and reasoned decision-making and has led to dissatisfaction from the medical profession, NHS ancillaries and the consumer alike.

NHS management developments of the last decade have neither prevented health policy continuing to be characterized by uncertainty and contradiction nor established any significant objectives for improvement of overall health status. Matters eventually reached a critical point in 1987/8 when financial constraints had led to very apparent cuts-backs in hospital services and a number of influential reports were published which lent support to the view that there had been 'a legacy of underinvestment in health care' (Griggs, 1990). In January 1988 widespread unease prompted the announcement of a review of the NHS which subsequently formed the basis of the most fundamental reform of the system since its beginnings in 1948.

The following chapters examine, from the perspective of public law, some of the more major concerns about recent developments and reform in health care provision and will seek to offer at least a partial explanation as to why the NHS has failed to fully realize its potential. Despite the concept of accountability forming the cornerstone of the initial ideals and organization of NHS, substantial problems of regulation and of the answerability of politicians, managers and medical professionals to the public are apparent. It will be suggested that diagnosis of the ills of the NHS has been deficient. Unless fresh consideration is given to the nature of the incorporation of accountability measures in the legislative and institutional framework of health care services difficulties are likely to recur.

The central argument is that insufficient attention has been given to the potential role of law in the shaping of health policy and the management of health services as a public organization. This first chapter concentrates on the relationship between law and policy and public management and lays the foundation for development of the main theme in subsequent chapters.

LAW AND POLICY

Essentially health care provision is rationed, hard policy choices have to be made about the selection of priorities, the allocation of resources and the availability of services. Inevitably, trade-offs continually have to be made between costs, quality and access which help expose weaknesses in the delivery and provision of services and give rise to doubts about the nature of policy decisions throughout the entire organization.

Debate about this latter, emergent problem is usually left to political scientists. With a few notable exceptions lawyers have made little contribution to discussion of general policy processes in the United Kingdom (Harden and Lewis, 1986). This is perhaps surprising as one of the key functions of law in society is to provide a framework for the conduct of public affairs. Law is one of the major means by which institutions such as those which provide health care, education or welfare benefits are established, defined and structured (Cotterall and Bercusson, 1988). Law is also frequently made and interpreted within those institutions by officers, managers or administrators during the processes of policy making and implementation. The reason for this is that statutory frameworks are of necessity for the most part merely enabling legislation which only broadly outline policy objectives and leave the detail of service provision to the exercise of delegated discretionary powers. Law therefore has both constraining and facilitative qualities and is an instrument for achieving public ends by the shaping of social processes.

What is perhaps under-emphasized is that law is not just, as described, an instrument for achieving goals but is also a means of promoting and ensuring accountability and legitimacy in public decision-making, principles which are fundamental to our ideas of democracy and citizenship. Although discretionary powers are a necessary feature of modern government, enabling public bodies to cope with changing circumstances with a degree of flexibility, our concepts of democracy and justice require that such powers are neither abused nor exercised unfairly.

Procedures for accountability help ensure that arbitrary decisions are eliminated and that policy is made for reasons that are properly related to the objectives of the grant of discretionary power. However, it is now widely recognized by constitutional commentators that present procedures for accountability through traditional democratic parliamentary processes, although supplemented and improved to some extent in recent years, fall far short of meeting modern demands for machinery that responds effectively to public policy needs. Yet legal theory is still in many ways attempting to come to terms with the failure of these traditional forms of law to deal with the current crises of accountability and legitimacy that are arising in many of our public institutions and the growing recognition that the statutory framework of an organization no longer corresponds in any direct way to the development and implementation of public policy (Prosser, 1982, 1986). Thus the formal structure of a public institution such as the NHS does not necessarily give any real indication of how decisional processes and machinery for accountability actually operate within it.

Where traditional means of securing fundamental, democratic ideals prove inadequate it follows that renewed consideration ought to be given to other ways of perfecting arrangements for their realization. In public institutions any fresh transfusion of means to revitalize democratic principles should seek to optimize opportunities for effective scrutiny and input into administrative or management processes for priority setting and resource allocation from those most affected.

Health care provision is no exception to the general situation described above. It need hardly be stated that this is an area of decision-making that is of immense social, economic and political relevance. It concerns the interests and limitations of public control over the allocation and utilization of public resources, and yet in the UK these matters have been exposed only to minimal public debate.

In the traditional sense, ultimate responsibility for the NHS lies with the Secretary of State who is directly accountable to Parliament through the usual processes of parliamentary questions, the Public Accounts Committee and the Select Committees on Social Services and now Health. But the extent of discretionary power means that to a considerable degree much decision-making in the NHS operates well outside the traditional machinery for democratic accountability.

Although the NHS is one of the most pervasive of all public services and a major contributor to decision-making which seemingly touches everyone at some time in their lives, health policy is an area which has been particularly devoid of attention by public lawyers (Parkin, 1985). Analysis by them has been mainly peripheral, focal points for law and health have been mostly concerned with liability for personal injury, medico-ethical issues and forensic matters. Whilst the concept of accountability for health policy has always been implicit in the organizational framework of the NHS, 'health law' has only rarely focused on the justifications for the provision and allocation of services under the public financing and regulation of the system. However, lawyers have a fundamental role to play in the analysis and development of the operation of our institutions as management of public organizations in general becomes more invasive and complex and the instantiation of accountability for policy decisions becomes increasingly problematic. This is particularly so in the highly specialized organization of the NHS, where accountability is a particularly shadowy concept.

ACCOUNTABILITY AND THE LAW-JOBS; A HOLISTIC VIEW

Accountability within the public arena has always been perplexing, often comprising a complex, heterogeneous mix of fiscal, managerial, professional and public forms. However in a public organization it is arguable that all these guises are really just aspects of one form, public accountability, as all the former can contribute in some way to the realization of the latter and hence to the legitimacy of decision-making of the whole.

Within the health service accountability is particularly tenuous, its multi-faceted and unbalanced aspects have not for the most part been fully recognized or at least have passed virtually unremarked on. Policy formation and implementation in the NHS are effected through extremely complex processes involving a wide variety of participants and influences. Bare description of the statutory and administrative structure of the NHS merely serves to understate the complexity and opacity of its decisional processes and does little to reveal the explanations or justifications for decisions. The problems which beset decision-makers in an organization where policy-making and execution may be influenced by so many factions therefore also remain unhighlighted. At many points within the national health system decisions about the allocation of resources and the provision of services may be crucially affected by those who have access to policy processes. Yet it is far from easy to map out the relative significance and shifting patterns of impact of the organization's constituent groups (politicians, civil service, health authority members and managers, the medical professions and ancillaries and of course 'the consumer'); not to mention any external pressures, from the medical supply or pharmaceutical industries for example.

These matters concern the sharing of public power amongst government in its broadest sense and other strategic groups and should be of considerable importance to public lawyers, posing for them questions of accountability which are antecedent to the drawing up of any effective organizational design. How are decisions made? By whom? What criteria are used? How are differences of purpose and influence negotiated and resolved? Are the ways and means to achieve objectives effective? Are all these processes properly monitored?

Within the context of the NHS Klein advocated a far more open, user responsive service when he suggested that accountability should mean:

> the acceptance of the responsibility publicly to explain and justify policies, to welcome rather than stifle discussion of priorities and objectives, awareness of and sensitivity to public needs and a willingness to remedy errors.
>
> (Klein, 1974, p. 365)

In terms of policy processes accountability has both *ex ante* and *ex post* elements, meaning that decisions not only need to be justified and open to challenge after they have been taken but, to ensure that the values reflected are those of the people most affected, machinery must be provided to allow involvement of relevant parties in policy processes at a stage before decisions become irrevocable.

The central prerequisite for genuine accountability is clearly openness, a transparency which needs to embrace all decision making from policy setting, through implementation to monitoring. A commitment to openness is of prime importance in order to counteract any tendency to control or distort information which might in turn prevent issues being the subject of proper debate and reduce capacity for reasoned choices to be made about priorities and resource distribution. This means that more than a basic provision for access to information is needed. To be successful openness requires the devising of mechanisms for the actual generation of information and its utilization, in order to widen policy options. The same commitment also implies an obligation on the part of decision-makers to give explanations and justifications for their activities. The articulation of reasons for action or inaction is beneficial to accountability in several ways. It not only assists the development of standards and principles, but encourages more care and deliberation on the purposes of action by decision-makers and also provides a basis for criticism and facilitates challenge to decisions which appear arbitrary (Galligan, 1982).

The main pursuit for lawyers is to actively assist in the development of procedures which seek to infuse these broad and far-reaching expectations of accountability into our public, organizational structures. It is only through properly responsive processes of accountability that a clear picture can emerge, that any defects can be made apparent and the changing patterns of alliances highlighted. In this way an opportunity can be provided for different views and interests to be brought to bear on practice and ultimately facilitate change.

Questions of accountability are therefore closely linked to issues of effectiveness and efficiency. Both are without doubt essential concerns in any enterprise, but they are complex and ambiguous concepts whose determination, as will be discussed later, is particularly problematic within health care provision. Put simply, effectiveness is an evaluative measure, it concerns the attainment of intended objectives and the quality of outcomes. It is quite different in nature to efficiency with which it is sometimes subsumed. Efficiency concerns the optimum use of resources and the maximization of output in relation to cost. Efficiency cannot be properly judged unless the criteria for effectiveness and quality are known. Hence, efficiency is subordinate to effectiveness and accountability is logically an indispensable precondition for the advancement of both (Birkinshaw *et al.*, 1990).

Latterly, however, the emphasis of the management of public institutions has been on efficiency, especially economic efficiency. A misconception appears to have arisen amongst public management that the requirements of wider, public accountability are either irrelevant to or are a constraint on its attainment (Ranson and Stewart, 1989). But the process of institutional reform is unlikely to be successful if guided only by instrumental rather than evaluative considerations. Truly effective and hence efficient action by any organization requires a capacity to learn through its arrangements for the setting and revising of objectives and policies and the monitoring of performance. Such arrangements constitute its procedures for accountability in all its different guises; the examination of which assists the learning process by the recognition of any real and potential differences in perceptions of objectives and of competing priorities throughout an institutions networks and initiatives.

Accordingly, accountability is inherently evaluative, its processes are the means by which the effectiveness of an institution may be judged and ultimately the means by which legitimacy is lent to its conduct. Accountability is also by nature dynamic, providing a vehicle for improvement. Without accountability techniques for performance review and organizational assessment, the search for effectiveness and quality is likely to be impeded. The hallmark of an accountable public service is thus one which properly and openly plans and evaluates services, monitors grievances and in doing so creates and maintains an institutional record of legitimate decision-making.

The issues just described are ones which are present to a greater or lesser extent in any organization. One of the most comprehensive and rational considerations of the requirements for their resolution was that put forward by Karl Llewellyn (Llewellyn, 1940). He argued that in order for any group or institution 'from a scout troop to the United Nations' to sustain stability and cohesiveness and thus function effectively a series of socially necessary tasks have to be performed (Harden and Lewis, 1984, p. 2). These interlinked and fundamental jobs do not promote the adoption of any specific organizational or procedural arrangements as these will be shaped by the context within which they are to operate, but they do provide a blueprint for collective activity.

There are four main concerns which Llewellyn called the law-jobs, which can provide the essential patents for shaping and adapting processes for the exercise of public power within the framework of modern policy making (see particularly Lewis, 1981).

GOAL ORIENTATION

The first job is that of choosing goals and objectives. This is concerned with the setting of priorities and development of policy. Within health care disparities in the allocation of resources can lead to injustice and unequal opportunity in the receipt of care. This means that health policy needs to be continually reassessed as information becomes available about the possibilities for improving overall health status, prophylactic measures and the facilities for care. These are essentially political decisions and the means for taking them need to be embodied in the structure of the system to ensure legitimacy.

THE CONSTITUTION OF GROUPS

This leads to the second law-job, that of the allocation of decision-making authority. The question of who is competent and who should have the power to take decisions is crucial to the legitimacy and effectiveness of an organization. It involves the structural and administrative framework within which the other tasks are carried out. This law-job is one which therefore brings into focus the exercise and control of delegated and discretionary powers and within the health service raises questions of the balance of authority and responsibility for the utilization of resources between management and clinicians.

PREVENTIVE CHANELLING

The third job for law is that of implementing policy and monitoring operations to ensure that chosen objectives are achieved. Monitoring is increasingly significant and evident in the processes of modern public administration and is especially apparent in recent developments within the NHS. Monitoring may be either internal or external and is necessary for both the recognition and avoidance of disputes. It is here where 'contemporary expressions of concern for legitimacy' and opportunities for wider constituencies to take part in policy processes can be implanted (Harden and Lewis, 1986, p. 68).

THE DISPOSITION OF THE TROUBLE CASE

The final law-job is that of resolving disputes and concerns the redress of all grievances relating to the system; matters which are crucial to questions of legitimacy and accountability. Although individually a dispute or complaint may not pose any threat to the stability and cohesion of a society or organization, accumulatively they may come to endanger the established order. Furthermore, grievance resolution can provide additional information and feedback of the system in operation and an effective channel of accountability.

In short, the law-jobs provide the conditions for genuine accountability of collective decisions through outlining the legitimate pattern of authority, the provision of information, and the machinery for policy making and the resolution of conflict. They thus help create a capacity for the public to obtain a clearer, wider and undistorted view of the operation and effectiveness of an organization. Law is perceived as a political resource that can be used to redesign social institutions to facilitate the coordination of action within and upon the system.

Within the UK the law-jobs are distributed throughout the legislative, judicial and administrative branches of government. But evidence of their existence is an unreliable and insufficient indicator that the potential of the law-jobs has been reached. The ideal of accountablity requires that we look very carefully at all the decision-making processes of the state to see if the law jobs are being fully realized. We must ask ourselves whether the way we get things done and the procedures that have been developed actually deliver what the law-jobs posit is constitutionally necessary for the stability, cohesion and maturity of our public organizations and of course ultimately for their legitimacy. If procedures are unacceptable or ineffective in delivering our desired ends we must look to see how they can be developed, revised or renewed so that they produce legitimate outcomes (Harden and Lewis, 1986, p. 69).

If the foregoing concept of law and its duties is applied to the provision of health care it can be seen that any discussion of the socio-economic problems of the NHS and its reform needs to be supported and broadened by examination of the organization's constitutional expectations and the arrangements which underpin them. This necessitates a close look at how the law-jobs are operating throughout the system and also an examination of the nature of management and the activities of managers and other networks and constituencies operating within it and upon it. Through such processes the extent to which the variety of potentially conflicting interests and policy outcomes are conditioned and accommodated by any systemic biases might be highlighted.

Thus an understanding of the institution's organization and the interconnections of its mechanisms for all its decisional functions are a precondition for actually releasing its capacity to operate in an effective and legitimate manner. Yet, an often neglected aspect of the 'revamping' of organizations is that in order to improve the quality and effectiveness of service, the quality of its organizational framework and the interplay of its many constituent actors also needs to be evaluated.

PUBLIC MANAGEMENT

The difficulties which have arisen in relation to accountability are in many ways a manifestation of the complex network of relationships between politics, public law and public management. The main purpose of accountability processes is to maintain the standards of performance of the organization for which they are devised.

In a public institution this is part of the political process; public managers are expected to work within a framework that is intended to ensure that resources are properly used and that the discretionary powers which are granted to managers to enable them to carry out their tasks are exercised for legitimate purposes. Accountability can therefore be said to be central to management concerns and responsibilities (Metcalfe and Richards, 1987, pp. 42–50). Superficially this may appear to be straightforward but in reality management of public organizations has raised a multitude of conceptual and practical difficulties. Just as there is a deal of debate and some confusion about what is meant by law and accountability there are similar difficulties in defining public management and specifying the responsibilities of public managers.

It is clear that the optimization of accountability of an institution and any consequent improvements in overall performance relating to quality, effectiveness and efficiency are allied to the promotion of better means of management. But this still begs the question, what is meant by public management? What does it entail? Sparse consideration appears to have been given to this by government when reforming public organizations in general and the NHS in particular, although perhaps political rhetoric would have us believe otherwise.

Instead, it has been assumed that public organization would benefit most from a closer alignment with the pattern and style of management of the private sector. However, it has been argued that this has resulted in an impoverished view being taken of public management by a denial of its distinctive features. Even though the focus of an organization is public it is often private management values that are accepted as the norm and many of the legitimate activities of a public body, particularly those related to public accountability become implicitly regarded as outside the concern of public management or are perceived as constraints on efficiency (Ranson and Stewart, 1989).

But the perceived incompatibility between public accountability and management is arguably more a consequence of a dissonance of forms and functions than of any inherent conceptual difficulty. It has already been argued that current, traditional processes of accountability are in many ways inadequate to meet the needs of modern state business. This is partly because they were designed long before such complex issues as quality, effectiveness and efficiency developed as legitimate concerns of modern public organizations and consequently the latter have little or no outlet in older established procedures (Metcalfe and Richards, 1987, p. 43). Instead, they have been introduced as 'part and parcel' of the private management techniques that have become assimilated into public management with very little consideration of devising more appropriate accountability measures.

In relation to the health services, as will be discussed later, there are specific difficulties in many areas which rule out any direct comparison between the responsibilities and activities of public and private managers.

The marginalization of the public features of public institutions has gone hand in hand with a marked trend towards the primacy of concerns for cost efficiency and 'value for money', both of which are management defined. Metcalfe and Richards point out that the inference is that these are politically neutral, '. . . a purely technical, instrumental means to politically approved ends . . . an unqualified good like apple pie or motherhood' (1987, p. 29). However, they go on to argue that the elevation of economic efficiency brings with it its own values which shape priorities and influence perceptions of problems as well as the feasibility of solutions. Thus the definition of what is significant in terms of economic efficiency means that concerns for effectiveness and quality may be downgraded such that they are considered to be standards which no longer have any independence from costs. Consequently, reliance on the technicism and instrumentality of economic efficiency can render accountability processes even more impotent as either checks on decision-making or guidance to policy.

The foregoing argument is not intended to deny that efficiency, effectiveness and quality may frequently be competing goals between which trade-offs have to be made. But public accountability requires that such trade-offs be made explicit. The current tendency to conflate all three factors into a concern for budgetary matters, particularly in an area such as health care where uncertain and changing factors may critically affect the public interest, means that policy is not the consequence of the open and reasoned decision-making that public accountability dictates should be the case.

That business orientation is the focus and that technology and economics are a present driving force of our public institutions is further evidenced by the trend towards what can broadly be called 'marketization'. This may take one or more forms of policy inter-vention such as privatization, changes in regulation, charging for services, the introduction of elements of competition through con-tracting out or internal tendering and contract arrangements. The rationale behind this trend is the belief that a pro-competitive market-orientation will improve efficiency, quality and account-ability by giving the public primacy, as individual consumers, in the market-place.

However, even though marketization may continue to become increasingly pervasive, the necessity for the conduct of government business is unlikely to diminish. Rather, the need for management of public matters is likely to increase through the introduction of varying forms for channelling government functions, concerns and interests and the diversity of public organizations, their interdepen-dence and networks of influence. In essence it can be argued that the introduction of elements of marketization to public organiz-ations merely redefines the requirements of both public manage-ment and public accountability (Metcalfe and Richards, 1987). The need for adaptive mechanisms of management and complementary, appropriate procedures of accountability are therefore in all prob-ability even stronger.

The health services in common with other areas of social policy have for some time been witnessing the introduction of private sector business practices and a pro-market orientation. This process began with the implementation of some of the recommendations of the Griffiths Inquiry into NHS Management (1983) and has con-tinued through subsequent reforms and changes which have intro-duced a series of commercial business practices and more latterly an element of competition through both internal and external con-tracting for the provision of services.

When a complex system such as the NHS has to respond rapidly to organizational changes and shifts in emphasis, priorities can be modified and decision-making criteria interpreted in ways that may not be in the best interests of the public. It is not the case that management merely implements policy that has been decided upon elsewhere; this view arises from too narrow a conception of management, and perhaps an unthorough understanding of policy processes.

Traditionally policy formation and policy implementation are regarded as distinct processes. But policy processes are much more interlaced and complex. Policy is rarely applied directly – it is mediated through institutions and those within them, so that the actual impact of policy is affected as much by these factors as by the merits of the policy itself. Even though central policy makers may attach reliance and significance on regulation and guidelines for policy, management and others involved in its execution will place their own construction on such advice and directives. Not only may policy be distorted or selectively interpreted from the 'top' down by the incorporation of the objectives and interests of different sections of an organization, but it may also be varied as a result of pressures and difficulties perceived from the ground (Dunsire, 1978; Dunleavy, 1980; Barrett and Hill, 1986; Metcalfe and Richards, 1987). Policy processes can be likened to the production of lace or webbing, the various strands of policy generating yet more detailed and intricate strands. In other words, differentiation between policy formation and implementation may be virtually indeterminable.

This has been as much a problem for the health service as any other organization, the supposed separation and lack of understanding of the nature of policy processes being liable to have an effect on both performance and accountability. In practice the recognition and realization of social values and public purposes has perhaps concentrated the minds and guided the activities of health service management less than the formal structure and policy initiatives of the organization imply. The tendency has been to concentrate on tangible, technical factors which are more readily measurable than more abstract objectives. The central concern that arises as a result of the latest reorganization is that public accountability should not be diminished to the point where a 'new élite structure, based on information, technical expertise, position and policy ideas comes to determine who gets what, when and why?' (Peters, 1978, p. 173).

CONCLUSION

Although several attempts have been made in recent years to improve the management of health-care provision, specifically in relation to containing costs, the tactics developed have added little to public knowledge of policy and resource allocation processes. Although openness and accountability are a fundamental requirement of any public institution and are in fact implicit in the organizational structure of the NHS, their realization is problematic and health care policy at all levels has tended to remain the result of tacit rather than explicit action.

It has been suggested in this chapter that an expanded concept of law may have a vital role to play in developing health care provision into a more legitimate and effectively managed service through the innovative design of procedures which seek to promote accountability by a better reflection of public choices and the provision of reasoned justifications for decisions. Such procedures could form a basis for the continual evaluation and improvement of our health care system and services. Thus, the development of procedures for the open planning and assessment of services and machinery which sought to elucidate the complex network of relationships which are part of the health care structure, the fulfilment of the law-jobs, would be the hallmark or 'chartermark' of an accountable NHS.

In the past as costs have become paramount the public accountability features of public institutions such as the NHS have been marginalized, but there needs now to be a recognition that a quality end product has a much higher potential for realization if the quality of decision-making processes are themselves reassessed in the light of the needs of legitimacy.

The following chapters seek to examine the extent to which the potential of the law-jobs is being fulfilled within our health care system, although on analysis of any organization it is difficult to separate out their various functions because they are inherently interlinked and operate symbiotically. Chapter 2 looks primarily at the first two law-jobs, namely goal orientation and the constitution of groups, Chapter 3 concentrates on policy management and the monitoring of services and Chapter 4 examines the disposition of 'the trouble case'. Chapter 5 then takes an overview of public accountability in recent 'market' and potential future developments. Finally in Chapter 6 the various strands of the argument are drawn together and the implications for public management, the role of law and accountability in the NHS are set out.

2

PRESCRIPTIVE DILEMMAS: ACCOUNTABILITY AND THE STATUTORY AND ADMINISTRATIVE STRUCTURE OF THE NHS

This chapter looks at how the first two law-jobs, namely goal orientation and the constitution of groups, operate within the NHS although inevitably implementation of policy will be touched upon. The structures for the setting of priorities and the development of health policy at central and local level are critically considered and questions of competency and the allocation of decision-making authority are raised. These are concerns which are crucial to the legitimacy of health policy and effectiveness of its delivery.

The statutory and administrative framework of the NHS is intended to facilitate the considerable complexities of translating broad objectives into operation at a local level and of turning resources into services. It follows a pattern familiar to both public lawyers and public management in that substantive aims and powers are stated only in very general terms and their implementation is left to the relatively unstructured discretion of the Secretary of State, the Department of Health in its several manifestations and the various health authorities. The two major re-organizations prior to the present one did little to alter this structure, nor at first sight do the latest reforms appear to depart radically from the traditional format. However some of the changes, particularly those at the lower end of the NHS hierarchy, could, if fully implemented, have unprecedented implications for future organizational coalitions and the balance of power within the system.

Together with the National Health Service Act 1977, which remains the principal Act, and the Health Services Act 1980, the National Health Service and Community Care Act 1990 (referred to as the 1990 Act from now on) provides the Secretary of State for Health with extremely broad and extensive discretionary powers. In practice however there is only a limited capacity for the exercise of any individual influence on health care decisions. The range and complexities of issues involved in running health services, not to mention the difficulties presented by the peripatetic nature of most Ministers' jobs, necessitate the majority of the Secretary of State's powers and duties being put into effect through the Department of Health, the NHS Policy Board, Management Executive, the health authorities and the recently established NHS Trusts.

The paramount power of the Secretary of State is that of controlling NHS expenditure through the use of cash limits. The total amount of funding annually available to the NHS each year is determined by the Public Expenditure Survey (PES) process and depends on the relative priority given to it by government and the demands of other departments. Since 1977 this amount was usually subdivided and allocated to health authorities on the basis of the Resource Allocation Working Party (RAWP) formula which sought to identify the health care needs of each regional population. Regional Health Authorities (RHA) tended to vary in the extent to which they then relied on the formula to allocate funds to their districts and in recent years funds were more likely to be distributed on the basis of planned service developments (*Working for Patients*, 1989, para. 4.5).

The RAWP formula was devised at a time when there was expected to be continuing increases in funding and was intended to make the distribution of resources more equitable. But it came to be applied in a period of financial constraint which meant, paradoxically, that gains could only be made for some districts at the expense of losses for others (Klein, 1989, p. 234). The overall result was that there was often no direct correlation between the amount of money a district was allocated and the number of patients it treated.

Since the financial year 1990–91 the use of the RAWP formula has been discontinued and a modified system of funding is being phased in. Health authorities will eventually be funded on a capitation basis, weighted to reflect the health and age distribution of the population and the relative cost of providing services. This process is expected to be completed by 1993/4 for regions and 1994/5 for most district health authorities. The new formulation is not, however, free of difficulties. A great deal of information about the composition of resident populations, their age and mortality rates needs to be known before the new system can be fully operational and as yet, adequate information is not readily available. Additionally, although one of the benefits of a population-based allocation scheme is that areas with fast-growing populations can be automatically compensated on an annual basis, the disadvantage is that districts with declining populations are likely to receive progressively less. Yet some of these latter districts serve areas of social deprivation. If these factors are not effectively incorporated into calculations and funding is not carefully adjusted and monitored, the result could be a less than equitable distribution of resources.

The Secretary of State is empowered to issue directions to RHAs 'with respect to sums made to them' and regions may likewise issue directions to their respective districts and Family Health Service Authorities. Any health authority to whom such directions are given is under a duty to comply. Overall financial control of spending by health services and the distribution of funds therefore continues to be strictly controlled by the utilization of cash limits which have statutory force. The regulatory package makes it clear that ultimate control lies at the centre where both financial and legal sanctions are available for non-compliance, although in the past these have been brought rarely into use.

Much more in issue are the structures for accountability of delegated decision-making and policy functions throughout the organization of the NHS. Formally the Minister carries ultimate responsibility for the exercise of all health service powers through the traditional parliamentary processes of Question Time, the Public Accounts Committee and the Select Committees on Social Services, and now Health. Although the committees mentioned have carried out in-depth investigations and produced some excellent reports in recent years on expenditure and the provision of services, for reasons mentioned in the previous chapter their impact is often constrained by the institutional framework within which they operate. As a consequence their influence and their success as guarantors of public accountability is relatively marginal, effective only to the degree that their conclusions are consistent with government policy (Harden and Lewis, 1986, pp. 106–11).

Until 1989 the Department of Health was assisted by a Health Supervisory Board and the National Health Service Management Board. Neither of these had any statutory basis, but were established on the recommendation of the Griffiths Inquiry into NHS

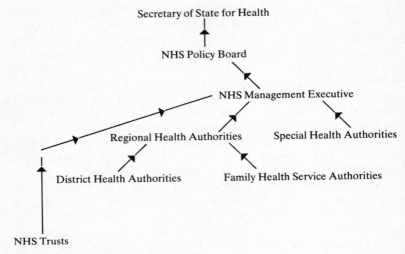

Figure 2.1   Statutory framework

Management (1983) in an attempt to improve central management and provide a rational framework for accountability between the Secretary of State and the Department of Health on the one hand and health authorities on the other. The Supervisory Board was set up as a strategic body which was to determine priorities, objectives and policy. The role of the Management Board was intended to be one of overall management, ensuring policy implementation. In practice, as perhaps might be expected following the difficulties of separating policy and implementation, the delineation of the respective roles and responsibilities of these two bodies was unclear. The Supervisory Board failed to become established as the central strategic force and eventually became defunct, whilst the functions of the Management Board became increasingly multi-faceted, due in part to the combination within it of civil servants and health service executive management.

Health authorities had assumed that the establishment of the Management Board indicated the introduction of a degree of autonomy from government control, but the civil service, perhaps not least because the Board came to be chaired by the Secretary of State for Health, appeared to regard the Board as a means to enhance direction of health service management (Stowe, 1988). The overall effect of these developments was a blurring of the lines

NHS Policy Board

Chairman – Secretary of State for
   Health
Chief Medical Officer
Chief Nursing Officer
Minister for Health
Parliamentary Under Secretary for
   Health (Commons)
Parliamentary Under Secretary for
   Health (Lords)
Permanent Secretary
Chief Executive of NHS ME
Plus seven non-executive members

NHS Management Executive

Chief Executive
Deputy Chief Executive – Director
   of Performance Management
Director of Health Care
Director of Nursing
Director of Corporate Affairs
Director of Finance and Corporate
   Information
Director of Research and
   Development
Director of Pensions

Figure 2.2

of accountability and management so that there was too much
involvement at the centre in detailed operational matters and
relatively less in the monitoring of policy implementation and its
effectiveness.

In an attempt to overcome these difficulties, NHS objectives,
strategy and finance are now determined, in the light of government
policy, by a National Health Service Policy Board. Central responsibility for operation and management of the health service
falls to the NHS Management Executive (NHSME), a branch of the
Department of Health whose remit is to work within the framework
set by the Department of Health and the Policy Board (Figure 2.1).

The Policy Board is chaired by the Secretary of State for Health
and operates with a rolling programme and meets about 10 times a
year. In order to bring a wide perspective to the formulation of
policy objectives for the NHS, members have been drawn from
government, the health service and industry and commerce (Figure
2.2). Although the non-executive members have been appointed
for their known support of government health policy it is a mix of
personnel and cultures which may itself in time produce some
bargaining complexities. The present 15 members are said to have a
strong commitment to their role and there is a strong bias towards
involving non-executive members in the Board's business.

The terms of reference of the Policy Board are to lend support to
ministers and to advise on the determination of strategy within
which the Management Executive will operate. The Board is also
expected to issue annual guidelines and set NHSME objectives
within available resources, monitor performance and comment

on the desirability and feasibility of specific goals proposed for the NHSME. The Policy Board itself draws on the advice and support of the divisions of the Department of Health, namely the Health and Social Services divisions (formerly the Policy Group) which have responsibility for the development of policies applied in and throughout the NHS. It is intended that the Board should be particularly concerned with the overall pattern and balance of policies for the NHS and with assessing the effectiveness of their implementation, rather than with the detailed formulation of specific policies. As the new system becomes established the Board's policy debates and the responses of health service central management need to be closely examined.

The functions of the Management Executive are:

- to issue strategic and operational guidelines to health authorities;
- to develop and advise the Policy Board of resource policies and needs;
- to propose the distribution of funds to the regions, and
- to deal with pay and personnel issues.

It also sets health authority targets and monitors their achievement through regional planning and review processes. The role of the NHS Management Executive now includes responsibility for primary care as well as acute and community health services.

Following a report by the then director of operations and planning which was critical of the structure of the Management Executive, the organization of the NHSME has now been streamlined in accordance with its core functions (Moore, 1991, p. 14). The report argued that although the executive was well designed to provide advice and support to ministers and to monitor the provision of health services, it was not particularly well designed to actually manage it. This of course reflects the differences in orientation between civil service and management perspectives of NHS organization and also mirrors the debates which have underpinned the development of 'Next Steps' agencies in other areas of government business (see Chapter 5).

In place of the previous eight directorates there are now seven (Figure 2.2). Only two directorates – research and development, and personnel – remain principally the same as before. The finance and corporate information directorates have been merged; and operations and planning, family health services and the medical division have been substantially reorganized. A health care directorate now brings together primary, secondary and community care, a merger to which the previous structure had been regarded as an obstacle. The corporate affairs directorate which defines the strategic framework of the NHS has taken over from operations and planning and a performance management directorate is now responsible for reviewing NHS performance. The intention is that this revised structure should overcome previous difficulties.

The NHSME meets bimonthly in its strategic mode and a great deal of reliance is placed on the personal accountability of the Chief Executive and the Directors. Besides being directly accountable to the Secretary of State the Chief Executive is the accounting officer for the Hospital and Community Services and Family Health Services and is expected to attend the Public Accounts Committee and other select committees as required. The performance of directorates must reflect objectives which are approved, checked and monitored by the Policy Board on a twice yearly basis. The Management Executive must submit to the Secretary of State and the Policy Board an annual plan rolled forward each year and an annual report, which includes health authority and FHSA outturn. At present the changes in culture within the Management Executive and the extension of exchanges of personnel between civil servants in the Department and management of the NHS are considered to be working well.

The NHSME is also satisfied that a clear role, that of implementing the reforms has now emerged for Regional General Managers. Although some regional functions have been devolved to district authorities the remit of Regional Health Authorities has been extended so that they have quite a formidable workload. RHAs are intended to concentrate their efforts on allocating financial resources, setting standards, monitoring and evaluating the effectiveness of health services in their region which include a string of additional functions which have come about as a result of changes to FHSA accountability. The eight or nine meetings a year between Regional General Managers and the Management Executive are regarded as the power house of strategic thinking and decisions taken at the annual conference of regional mangagement are fed through this meeting cycle.

Regional chairmen no longer have any management function but are regarded as 'the eyes and ears' of the Minister who is meant to maintain a distance from regional management. Regional chairmen have their own secretariat and meet every month and with the Minister every other month. Communication is also maintained between the Department of Health and the NHS through joint working parties and meetings with advisory groups and representative national bodies such as the National Association of Health Authorities and Trusts (NAHAT)(Ham, 1990).

In line with government policy to devolve as much decision-making as possible to a local level, the Chief Executive of the NHS Management Executive has stated that the flow of guidance to health authorities will be cut to an absolute minimum to allow general managers an opportunity to develop a 'high quality, cost effective service suited to each districts needs' (Nichol, 1989, p. 660). Whether this 'hands off' approach is actually likely to emerge in practice is questionable. Firstly, the focus on economic efficiency remains paramount, all levels of the organization are under an obligation to deliver an efficient service within predetermined resources and consequently must monitor lower level performance. The temptation to provide guidance and intervene at a prescriptive level will be high. Secondly the difficulties that have marked successive health service reorganizations in the past as a result of the somewhat artificial split between policy making and execution may not yet have been dealt with adequately.

Similar difficulties to those experienced in central management in relation to policy processes were evident within health authorities. In theory health authority members of both regional and district tiers had responsibility for formulating policies and taking strategic decisions, and the function of managers and staff was to advise and implement policy and oversee the day to day operation of services. In practice of course this differentiation was inevitably fudged and some overlap and interchangeability existed between the respective roles of the two groups. Health authorities came to be perceived by government as neither truly representative nor management bodies. An attempt has been made to resolve incompatibilities by placing increased reliance on business management skills and decreasing the community representation element. Changes have been made to the membership of health authorities, ostensibly on the grounds of an intention 'to extend responsibility for complex managerial and contractual issues to a local level' (*Working for Patients*, 1989, paras 8.3–8.5).

Each tier is now reduced to five non-executive members and up to five executive members, plus a non-executive chair. Chairs of both levels of health authorities and non-executive members of RHAs are appointed by the Secretary of State, and District Health Authority (DHA) non-executive members by the relevant RHA. Executive members include the general manager, financial director and others appointed by non-executive members. However, non-executive appointments are now made solely on the basis of the skills and experience members can bring to the work of the health authority, rather than for representation of any particular interest group. In the latest round of appointments this has led to an over-emphasis of members from the business community. A survey of 82 districts conducted by the British Medical Association found that out of more than 410 non-executive members 164 were from a business background and just 51 from the medical profession (*BMA News Review*, 1991).

The reduction of wider community representation and the loss by local authorities of their previous right to appoint members to DHAs is a cause for concern. If DHAs are to fulfil their role in identifying local needs and responding to the wishes of the resident population and planning services accordingly improved avenues for consultation and enhanced means of local representation need to be present. The arguments for retaining some local authority representation are forceful, as the job of the local authority representative can be significant in easing collaboration for the planning and financing of community services between health authorities, local authorities and the independent sector. And yet the BMA found that only 31 local councillors had been chosen as members. As will be discussed below, DHAs are in the process of building up alliances with other community agencies concerned with health care to fulfil their new functions, but these are discretionary and for the most part are being developed on an informal basis, with no regulatory framework to encourage systematic wider public input.

GENERAL PRACTICE

Since its inception a prominent feature of the NHS has been the separation of general practice from hospital services. General practitioners (GPs) are independent contractors who derive their income from a blend of various forms of payment. GPs operate a primary care service and some 90 per cent of general practice consultations are dealt with entirely within the practice. The remaining percentage are referred to hospital for further investigation, a second opinion or treatment. The general practitioner also therefore carries out what is commonly referred to as a 'gatekeeper function' in relation to acute services and has a key role to play in controlling access to hospital services and use of resources.

Since 1985 responsibility for the planning and management of general practitioner services has been that of the Family Health Service Authorities (FHSA), formerly the Family Practitioner Committees. As a result of the latest reorganization FHSAs have been given a number of additional tasks. These include oversight of the introduction of indicative prescribing amounts for general practitioners, GP practice budgets, medical audit, and the development of information technology to assist the monitoring of GP prescribing and referral rates. As a consequence of its extended role certain changes have been made to FHSA structure, management and line of accountability.

The size of FHSAs has been slimmed down and each now has 11 members. The Chair is appointed by the Secretary of State. The other members, four of whom must be family health professionals, are appointed by the relevant RHA. General Managers have also been appointed to be responsible for the management of administrative business and the implementation of new FHSA responsibilities. Instead of being directly accountable to the Department of Health as was previously the case, FHSAs are now accountable to the relevant RHA which allocates FHSA funds, reviews performance and monitors their plans, which must be coordinated with those of the DHAs. This change in the line of accountability of FHSAs is a move which has been generally welcomed and should lead to better strategic integration of primary health care and hospital services. In order to discharge responsibilities with the degree of flexibility necessary for different areas FHSAs are free to determine their own sub-committee structures, with the exception of those committees which deal with complaints about practitioners who are allegedly in breach of their contract and the Medical Audit Advisory Committee.

In April 1990 the government introduced a new contract for general practitioners, although in essence this was more a modification of the previous one. The new contract aims to influence both the quality of care and costs. In line with the general ideology to stimulate 'consumerism' in the provision of health care there has been a small but important change in the way doctors' pay is calculated, in that capitation pay has been increased and the basic practice allowance decreased. There are also a number of measures which aim to relate financial awards to the quality of care:

● The use of deputizing services has been discouraged through the introduction differential pay for call out during unsocial hours.

- Targets have been set for some preventive measures such as childhood immunizations and cervical cytology.
- Payments will also be made for medical checks carried out on all new patients and those over 75 years of age.
- Any patients suffering from a chronic condition will attract additional payment.

GENERAL PRACTICE FUND HOLDERS

One of the more radical changes to health service provision at the lower end of the organization is the introduction of practice budgets for general practices. These measures are seen by government to provide an opportunity to improve the quality of services by stimulating competition for patients between general practitioners, and competition for contracts between general practices and district authorities.

Practices or groups of practices with at least 9000 patients are able to apply for budgets to purchase a defined range of hospital services such as outpatients services, diagnostic tests and some in-patient and day-case treatments, particularly those where there is some opportunity for choice about the time and place of treatment. Budgets also include allowances for practice costs, staff and premises and drugs. The element of the budget concerned with hospital services is deducted from the allocation of the relevant DHA. A current upper limit of £5000 has been placed on the cost of hospital treatment which a practice has to meet from its own budget for any individual patient. Perhaps surprisingly, RHAs rather than FHSAs are responsible for considering applications for funding and for determining the size of GP fund-holder budgets, despite the latter being required to be involved in the budget setting process because of their detailed local knowledge. The reason given by government for this was that FHSAs were considered to be too close to practitioners in their area. The provision does, however, to some extent maintain the philosophy of the separation of funding and provision, evident throughout other sectors of the service.

One of the main criticisms of practice budgets is that public confidence in GPs may be undermined and the present patient–doctor relationship distorted if financial considerations have to be taken into account in clinical decisions. The concern is that budgets may place doctors in the unwelcome position of having to seek savings from patient medical care to fund other developments in their practices and consequently may avoid taking on relatively costly patients such as the elderly or those with chronic disease. When questioned on this point by the Social Services Select Committee the Secretary of State replied that this would not be allowed to happen since specific local needs of patients would be taken into account when practice budgets are set (Social Services Committee, 1989, p. 19). However, this may be insufficient to reduce the risks of funded practices favouring healthy patients. A number of complaints that GPs are unwilling to take on patients with a chronic condition which requires continual prescribing have already been received by FHSAs (Longley, 1992).

Other criticisms focus on the efficacy of operating practice budgets. A patient population of 9000 is regarded by some to be too low to make allowances for any risk of high cost incidents without distorting available resources. Enthoven suggested that a viable patient population, one that could absorb risk, should have between 50 000 and 100 000 patients (Enthoven, 1989, p. 1167). In addition there is frequently a lack of the managerial skills and information technology necessary to run budgets effectively. Not only are information systems either absent from general practices or inadequate for the enlarged tasks of fund holding, but health-care providers themselves do not yet generally have sufficiently detailed data available to enable GPs to make informed judgements about the quality and costs of the care which they seek to purchase. Although district health authorities have compiled information packs for commissioning GPs, at present these tend only to set out broad quality principles and list available services and the number of patients treated in each speciality.

Marinker points out, however, that many of the criticisms levelled at budgeted practices have previously been made about contemporary general practice. He argues that many aspects of budget holding are just extensions and elaborations of current practice. What is new and giving rise to concern is the scale and speed at which this is taking place (Bevan and Marinker, 1989, pp. 27–34). There appear to be few safeguards within the process to ensure that patients will benefit individually or that general practitioners will be accountable to the public for the operation of practices and services provided other than in relation to expenditure.

All practices will have to produce annual reports and the accounts of practice budgets will be audited by the Audit Commission for Local Authorities and National Health Service as part of its audit of

FHSA and RHA accounts. Regulations have been made which specify the categories of valid expenditure and also how surpluses may be spent. These are supplemented as necessary by detailed guidance. Even though there is no intention that surpluses should boost the individual income of doctors it will be very difficult to prove that this has not in fact occurred.

Further means to contain costs in general practice have been introduced through the use of allocated indicative amounts for drugs. Expenditure on drugs is the largest single element of family health services spending and an attempt to control wasteful and unnecessarily expensive prescribing was initiated by the Selected List in 1984. The new arrangements are intended to place 'a downward pressure on expenditure on drugs'. Indicative drug amounts – which include appliances, dressings and chemical reagents – are based on the average for practices in the area and are intended to encourage prescribing of generic drugs instead of expensive alternatives, and to discourage any prescribing at all where the benefit to patients would only be marginal.

GPs fear that the use of indicative drug amounts will lead to a loss of clinical freedom to prescribe and point out that the cost of medication should be viewed in terms of quality, effectiveness and efficiency. Older generic drugs are often less effective than continually developed, branded ones and sometimes carry considerable side-effects which affect the quality of a patient's well-being. These factors have long-term implications for the totality of costs for health care which should be carefully monitored so that open appropriate standards for quality, not only monetary costs, can be ascertained (Bevan and Marinker, 1989, pp. 13, 14).

NHS TRUSTS

The culmination of the devolution of management responsibility and decision-making to a local level is the provision in the 1990 Act for the establishment of NHS Trusts as separate legal entities within the NHS, but outside health authority management structure. Any NHS unit actively involved in patient care may apply for Trust status. The definition of an NHS Trust is therefore flexible and may include hospitals, community-based services either alone or together with hospitals, ambulance services and even the provision side of DHAs. The management independence of NHS Trusts is intended to enable them to respond more effectively to patient needs and improve the quality of service:

> Whilst remaining fully within the NHS, Trusts differ in one fundamental respect from district managed units – they are operationally independent. Trusts have the power to make their own decisions – right or wrong! – without being subject to bureaucratic procedures, processes or pressure from higher tiers of management.
>
> (*Working for Patients. NHS Trusts; A Working Guide*,
> 1990, p. 2)

Encouraging the establishment of NHS Trusts is seen by government as a means of 'securing a commitment to the local community and encouraging local pride'.

In addition to the general powers held by establishments within DHA management, Trusts have extensive powers to acquire, own and dispose of assets; borrow subject to an annual limit; build up reserves; set their own management structures; employ and direct their own staff; and determine pay and conditions of service. Trusts are to 'compete' for business and earn their revenue from the services they provide. The main source of income will come from contracts with DHAs for the provision of care to residents. Other contracts and revenue will come from GP groups who hold their own budgets and other health authorities, as well as the private health care sector.

Hospitals or other facilities which are considering Trust status are first required to register 'an expression of interest' by sending an outline of their plans detailing the hospitals or units which will make up the Trust and the services it will provide, together with details of proposers. No hard and fast rules about the configuration of Trusts has been laid down by the government to allow maximum flexibility, but the following factors are taken into account: size and adaptability, existing integration, patient choice and competition, the effect on purchasing and local views.

Trusts are statutory corporations, run by their own board of directors, who have responsibility for determining overall policy, monitoring implementation and maintaining the financial viability of the Trust. The board consists of a non-executive chairman appointed by the Secretary of State, up to five non-executive directors, two of whom are to be drawn from the local community. 'Local directors' are appointed by the RHA, the remainder by the Secretary of State. Where a Trust has a significant commitment to undergraduate medical teaching one non-executive director must be drawn from the relevant university. Chairmen and non-executive members are appointed for periods of up to four years and in contrast to non-executive members of health authorities receive remuneration. Some groups who may have some knowledge of health service activities are not eligible for appointment as non-executive directors including GPs and their employees, members and employees of health authorities and other health service bodies and employees of trade unions with members who work in the NHS. This provision seems surprising, but is presumably an attempt to deter potential clashes of interest.

There must also be on the board an equal number of executive directors including the chief executive, the director of finance and for the majority of Trusts a medical and a nursing director. Directors are not personally liable for the actions of the board, otherwise their legal status is uncertain (Jacob, 1991). Apart from these requirements at board level, Trusts are free to develop management arrangements tailored to their needs.

Trusts are accountable to the Health Secretary via the NHS Management Executive and are subject to legislation that applies directly to NHS facilities such as the Hospital Complaints Procedure Act 1985, the Data Protection Act 1984 and the Access to Health Records Act 1990. In addition trusts are expected to take account, amongst others, of relevant EC directives; the requirements of statutory bodies, advice relating to patient, public or staff safety, personal privacy and patient confidentiality. However, except in relation to grievance handling and arrangements for communicable diseases, instructions and guidance issued by the NHS Management Executive will not normally apply to NHS Trusts. Unless otherwise directed by the Secretary of State, Trusts have a discretion whether to follow such guidance. Like health authorities Trusts are not Crown bodies and do not benefit from Crown immunity.

There are three main accountability measures which apply to Trusts although their effectiveness as far as overall public accountability is concerned is questionable, since, as might be expected requirements concentrate mainly on fiscal matters. Trusts are required to produce an annual business plan, in which it is expected to set out plans to develop services, financial projections and capital building plans. This is not a public document. However, the annual report of the previous year's performance and accounts is available for public perusal. Trusts are also required to provide in-year financial monitoring information, a 'small core of statistical data necessary to support Ministers public accountability for the NHS as a whole', information on capital schemes requiring Management Executive or Treasury approval and annual reports under the AIDS (Control) Act 1987. They must also inform the Management Executive if their long-term financial viability is at risk. Trusts are under a statutory duty to break even taking one year on another and are required to achieve a 6 per cent return on assets and keep within their agreed External Financing Limit.

The legal position of these new institutions is interesting. The term NHS Trust is a term of art which was substituted for the earlier one of self-governing hospital. Trust has symbolic advantages over its predecessor, in that to some extent it undermines the assertion that such institutions were 'opting out' of the NHS and at the same time manages to convey the impression they operate for the benefit of the public and not for any profit motive (Hughes, 1991). NHS Trusts are certainly not trusts in the usual legal sense as they fail to fulfil the necessary legal requirements for that status and are subject to a degree of executive control that no ordinary trusts experience. It is unlikely that any significance will be attached to Trust terminology or any analogy to true trusts will be applied by the courts. Instead, Trusts, like health authorities, are more probably to be regarded as public bodies for the purposes of judicial review.

PUBLIC PARTICIPATION IN HEALTH CARE POLICY

Community Health Councils (CHCs)

As the structure of the NHS in recent years has become increasingly concerned with management review and accountability for expenditure, dissatisfaction has often been expressed, despite the setting up of CHCs, with the consistent failure to foster measures for a wider concept of public accountability and facilitate adequate consumer input and representation.

Community Health Councils were established in 1974 and are under a broadly defined statutory duty to represent the public in their district (NHS Act 1977 Sch 7 and CHC Regs 1985). Although CHCs have been criticized for not being generally representative of the local community because of the preponderance of members from the professional sections of society they do go some way to providing a systematic element of public involvement in health matters at a local level. About half of the 18–24 members are nominated by the local authority, although nominees need not be councillors, a third by local voluntary organizations and the remainder by the RHA. The term of service is usually four years and each CHC has a Chairman and Vice-Chairman chosen by the members. Paid support staff is minimal but usually includes an Adminstrator who is employed by the Regional Authority, but who is chosen by and is accountable to the CHC, and a paid assistant, although the latter may vary between Councils. The financial budget of CHCs is agreed with the relevant RHA and covers the cost of staff, premises and running expenses.

There has always been a lack of guidance on how CHCs should fulfil their function and each Council has had to interpret and negotiate its own working relationship, not only with its DHA but with other institutions concerned with health care and with the consumers CHCs are designated to represent. This has inevitably resulted in some diversity of CHC involvement and effectiveness in local planning (Klein and Lewis, 1976, pp. 124–6).

Although under the current reorganization the statutory duties of CHCs remain unaltered subsequent guidance has introduced a number of key changes which affect CHC involvement in local health planning (EL (90) 185). CHCs have a right to be consulted by the relevant DHA when a substantial development or variation in services is contemplated. There are no provisions for CHCs to be consulted on health care issues on a wider, regional or national basis although some RHAs do, on occasion, involve CHCs in strategic planning; and the Association of Community Health Councils in England and Wales (ACHCEW) regularly considers and submits responses to national policy documents to the Department of Health and the NHS Management Executive (Hogg, 1986).

On the face of it, the provision for consultation suggests that there is an underlying intention that decisions should be subject to open and reasoned debate to enable differing interests to be taken into account before policy has become consolidated and that coherent and defensible reasons for action or non-action will be put forward. Consultation procedures thus imply a commitment to *ex ante* accountability. But in practice consultation more frequently results in a process of exclusion rather than inclusion because of differential access to information and resources which enables preferred groups to set agendas and the terms of debate before the consultation process begins in earnest (Harden and Lewis, 1986). The process of consultation, if not carefully structured and monitored, may therefore simply perform a legitimizing function rather than provide a channel for any real contribution to decision-making.

Several criticisms of CHC consultation procedures in particular and health service consultation provision generally can be made on this account. The process of consultation in relation to a variation in services is generally two staged. Initially there is a period of informal consultation on tentative, though often well-advanced, proposals. Generally this amounts to no more than a definition of the issues by exchange of letters or low-key discussion at an informal meeting. There then follows a short period of formal consultation in which comments are invited within three months (ACHCEW, 1986). It is suggested in Department of Health guidelines that the consultation document should set out, amongst other things, the reasons for change, the relationship with other development plans and implications for patients. The guidelines envisage that where sufficient local agreement exists it should be possible to move from proposal to actual implementation within six months (HSC(IS)207). However, there is no requirement for the health authority to publish its response to any CHC comment or to give reasons for rejection of any proposals put forward by the CHC.

CHCs have never been empowered to enforce any recommendations they might make and could only veto proposed changes in service provision if able to put forward a viable alternative that was accepted by the health authority. When responding to consultation CHCs are now no longer required to submit any counter-proposal, but a frequent complaint of health councils remains that they receive insufficient information about proposed changes, making both rational comment and the task of even suggesting that there are any acceptable alternatives extremely difficult (Birkinshaw, 1985).

Temporary or phased changes in provision generally lie outside the above procedures and some health authorities have evaded consultation by labelling changes as temporary even though the Department of Health guidelines concede that temporary changes can result in 'a substantial variation' of services and should not then be exempt from consultation processes. There is no definition of either 'temporary' or 'substantial' in legislative provisions and several disputed variations in service have given rise to applications for judicial review where it has been alleged that consultation requirements have not been fully complied with. However, litigation has so far failed to bring about any revision of either guidelines or actual consultation procedures, with the result that the influence of CHCs on service variations tends only to be marginal and rearguard, despite taking up a disproportionate amount of health councils' resources and time. Further restraint is placed on CHC effectiveness by their being unable to take legal action on their own behalf or on behalf of those they represent. In future, it is the health authorities themselves who are to determine what is to be considered a 'substantial variation' in the use of hospital buildings or the closure of services for the purposes of consultation.

Where consultation is carried out the time allowed may be far too short to enable a thorough examination of all the issues; this is aggravated by the fact that plans may be changed without allowing for further examination and comment. Any need to submit all comments received on proposed changes to the relevant CHC for a final response has been dropped. There is no obligation to repeat the consultation process unless any revised proposals are so different that they constitute fresh proposals. The question whether the revised proposals are sufficiently different to warrant fresh consultation is essentially a matter of degree (R v Shropshire Health Authority *ex parte* Duffus 1989). Nor is there any obligation to consult where the DHA is satisfied that in the interest of the health service a decision has to be taken without allowing time for consultation (1985 Regs para 19(2)).

Although an appeal lies to the relevant RHA where district management has failed to provide information or undertake consultation, there is no statutory provision for appeal to the Secretary of State from a decision of a health authority to vary services.

NHS Trust Applications

Of equal concern are consultation requirements for applications for Trust status. Such applications are subject to statutory public consultation which is undertaken by regional authorities who then report the results to the Secretary of State (1990 Act s5.) There is a duty to consult the CHC for the district in which the Trust is to be located and other bodies whom RHAs consider to have an interest in the application or are directed to consult by the Health Minister. Those consulted are likely to vary according to the nature of the Trust, but in addition to CHCs, guidance suggests the inclusion of relevant health authorities and FHSAs, staff in the proposed Trust, local GPs, the local community and local MPs. The government has stated that it is important that Trust applications are given wide publicity to ensure that all those who wish to make their views known have the opportunity to do so (*Working for Patients. NHS Trusts; A Working Guide*, 1990, p. 42).

However, meaningful consultation is reliant on the supply of sufficient information and mechanisms which are adequate to ensure that relevant views have been taken into account. Similar criticisms to those made in regard to substantial variations in health services can be made of Trust consultation processes. The period for consultation is again only three months, a short time for a considered response to what are often only basic details and from which financial details are omitted. Public meetings are left to the discretion of RHAs and Trust applicants and the organization of ballots is specifically excluded from the consultation process. The reason given for this was that ballots are thought unlikely to assist the Secretary of State in assessing the impact of the proposal on local services or the ability of management to run the proposed Trust. This contrasts sharply with consultation and ballot requirements for the opting out of schools from local education authority control under the Education (Reform) Act 1988. Under ss60, 61 of that Act a secret ballot of parents must be held and individuals have a right to object to the Minister if a proposal to 'opt out' of local authority control is forwarded to him. In addition the governing bodies of grant maintained schools must include a number of parent governors, to represent the consumer interest.

It is significant that it is not until after the business plan has been developed and the application prepared that any statutory provision for consultation is made. Consultation is therefore conducted well after plans have crystallized and a great deal of energy and resources have been expended. Amongst the eight key factors on which Trust applications are to focus in order to obtain the approval of the Secretary of State are the 'overall aims of the trust and the benefits for the patients and the local community' and 'the way in which services will be developed and quality assured'. These are obviously matters about which the public as consumers either individually or collectively might have an interest and might wish to express a view. It is also a matter of concern that Trusts are under no duty to consult CHCs if they are considering the closure of a unit or change in their activities.

The role of DHAs

The new role now being forged for district health authorities, that of 'champion of the people' (Developing Districts EL (90) MB/86) has significant implications for CHCs, and public consultation about policy as DHAs are being encouraged to develop links with local resident and community groups. The current changes in both the structure and function of DHAs could provide the opportunity to accommodate real consumer participation rather than mere rhetorical acknowledgement, and redress the balance between management, medical professions and consumers.

The 'consumer advocate' function of DHAs is providing a challenge which entails changes to DHA philosophy and culture, which many health authorities are doing their best to meet. But it is important to recognize that the means by which DHAs build up 'healthy alliances' could be crucial to the establishment of public input to health care planning and the future viability of both district authority and CHC roles. In the process of setting up community panels and forums it might be sensible and even necessary for DHAs to provide resources to CHCs so that the latter's skills, knowledge and expertise are neither duplicated nor lost. CHCs, although perhaps an imperfect player, should be allowed to play a key role in the development of a system which could aid the proper identification of shared interests and provide wider public input into policy.

Although the opportunity exists to ensure effective representation and appraisal of all relevant interests, much depends on health authorities being prepared to be innovative about devising arrangements and open in their conduct. In reality it will be extremely difficult for health authorities to adopt a role of reconciling the potentially varying views about what is needed for the locality. The development of alliances might mitigate the danger which some DHAs feel that as institutions they are likely to be vulnerable to criticism from all quarters and would undoubtedly have the advantage for the consumer of highlighting some of the informal decision-making networks which currently operate. But it requires a strong commitment to open decision-making and broadened access to requisite data. One of the key factors is to seek to ensure that information is available at a time and in a form that optimizes its usefulness. This is currently constrained by both managerial and governmental operational philosophy.

CONCLUSION

This chapter has been mainly descriptive in that it has examined the current administrative structure of the NHS. Inevitably, because many of the arrangements described are so recent and largely untested it has perhaps raised more questions than it has supplied answers about how policy decisions are made and the degrees of influence that the various contributors may have on policy processes. What is clearly arguable, however, is the need for empirical research into the implications of the responses to policy of all participant groups throughout the hierarchical structure, and a clearer consideration of the effects of the 'division' between policy formation and implementation. Once a comprehensive analysis has been made the lines of accountability should be clarified and the areas and processes requiring improvement highlighted.

It is also clear that the latest reforms have failed largely to grasp the opportunity to enhance participation in health policy by the public or their representatives, as statutory consultation measures remain minimal and for the most part ineffective; the classic case of 'too little, too late'. Additionally, the ' champion of the people' role which DHAs are being encouraged to espouse relies more on goodwill than clear, structural guidance.

Consequently, public effectiveness in countering managerial or health care provider perspectives and in participating in policy decisions is likely to continue to tend towards tokenism unless supported by an institutional framework that is procedurally structured to ensure that consumer interests are properly taken into account. Health care is without doubt a political issue in the true sense and any legitimate analysis of its provisions necessitates informed political and ethical discussion of all perspectives. In the past the public, through CHCs, have been allowed only limited scope to present their views. If an independent consumer voice is to function adequately in the post-1990 National Health Service – and it is argued here that some body independent of health authorities, at least whilst in their present form, should – then substantial changes have to be made as regards the powers, organization and available resources for consumer input. Such changes might then begin to enable the kind of informed, rational discourse implicit in democractic principles and the law-jobs.

3

CUTS, SUTURES AND COSTS: IMPLEMENTING POLICY AND MONITORING STANDARDS

This chapter examines primarily the third law-job, that of preventive channelling, the implementation and monitoring of policy in such a way as to ensure that chosen goals are attained. Monitoring may be both internal and external, but properly constituted and operated these processes have a potential to provide means for wider interests to have a role in policy decisions.

QUALITY

In recent years there has been a steadily increasing awareness of the need to monitor, appraise and review the quality of all public services. Although developments are fuelled largely by the desire to contain costs and attain value for money, major initiatives – launched by government to improve Civil Service management and management of public utilities – have produced some in-depth debate about indicators for assessing quality of service and consumer need (Pollitt, 1986). Within the health care field the difficulties of providing quality services are a major issue independent of the means of funding and delivery. The inevitable tension which exists between the attainment or maintenance of quality and fiscal issues give rise to legitimate and pressing matters which involve both financing processes and those of law.

Law has from very early times been concerned to assure the quality of care provided by the medical profession and the institutions in which they operate through accountability mechanisms such as malpractice cases, self-regulation or administrative codes and practices. The role of law in the process of quality assurance is required to be both varied and flexible in order to balance and facilitate such diverse goals as patient satisfaction, improved health outcomes and efficiency in health care delivery. Although quality assurance mechanisms are now an integral and often substantial part of the regulation of many health care systems, the organization of the NHS has generally been characterized by few such regulatory features. Progress in this area has been slow to get off the ground and it is only recently that the NHS has begun seriously to tackle the issues and means necessary for the monitoring and improvement of standards of quality.

As recently as 1988 the National Audit Office (NAO) criticized the Department of Health for failing to agree a national strategy for ensuring the quality of care. Performance indicators and annual planning and review processes have focused almost entirely on activity levels and resource use and have tended to neglect the more difficult dimensions of outcomes of care and input by consumers. Now that health authorities are expected to develop surer ways of assessing and measuring performance through means which include the extension of the Resource Management Initiative (RMI) and introduction of medical audit, certain questions need to be asked from the standpoint of the legal process and regulation. These include:

● To what extent and how can law assist to maintain standards of care?
● How can the tensions between cost containment and quality be best expressed in law?
● What guidance can law give to providers and purchasers attempting to balance financial concerns with the provision of high quality care? (Annas *et al.*, 1990, Chapter 5)

These questions are as complex as they are essential as the demand for health care expands and the provision of a high quality service from scarce resources becomes a priority.

Monitoring quality is a problematic process which needs to be carefully planned and requires a substantial investment in resources. A whole spectrum of quality issues exist which involve both individual and collective matters and which range from technical issues through the activities of the medical profession and management, where responsibilites and powers overlap, to the quality of outcomes. For effective quality assurance there are several essential tasks which need to be carried out (Jost, 1988). First of all the concept of quality for which evaluative techniques are being operated must be specified. Within health care there are five basic concepts of quality which are interlinked and inevitably tend to overlap, but which require different quality assessment and accountability processes.

The first of these is basically technical and is concerned with the reliability of facilities and equipment in meeting defined standards. The focus is the relatively stable characteristics of inputs, the tools and resources which providers have at their disposal and the organizational arrangements for the delivery of care, including arrangements for checking that facilities and equipment are used appropriately. These aspects of care are the easiest to define and evaluate and correlate closely to BS 5750 standard for quality management performance.

The second is concerned with professional competence, whether tests and treatment have been administered competently. The third and closely related concept is that of process which also concerns the activities of medical and other professionals in the provision of health care. It considers, for example, whether the appropriate diagnostic tests were made and whether the correct treatment was given or drug dosage prescribed. Process evaluation is usually based on current medical practice for any given problem and forms the basis of medical audit and peer review schemes. Process is less easy to evaluate than structure. Although it should be possible to correlate good quality and informed medical opinion there is often a lack of information about the efficacy of even well-accepted clinical procedures or incomplete or ambiguous evidence about the value of specific services, resulting in a wide variation in medical practices. Much work therefore needs to be done to develop and validate clinical practice before informed judgements can be made.

The fourth concept of quality is concerned with health outcomes, analysis here concentrates on the results of care and changes in the current and future health status that can be attributed to antecedent health care. Outcome analysis is the most difficult type of evaluation because the duration, timing and extent of outcomes often make optimal care hard to specify. In addition it requires the effects of medical care to be seen not only in the light of patients' own goals and weighing of risks and benefits, but to be distinguished from other factors such as personality or environmental matters.

Finally there is the concept of quality that is concerned with respect for personality rights which relate to the attitude and manner in which services are delivered; was there respect for privacy, was the patient kept informed? In order to clarify and utilize most beneficially the different concepts and interpretations of quality which might be applied by different constituencies a framework is required that can ensure ongoing co-operation and negotiation between all parties involved or affected by health delivery.

The second essential requirement for an effective quality assurance system is that it must be capable of setting standards, to define what these are in particular contexts. For example in order to differentiate between good and poor operative techniques or a good or poor intensive care unit it is necessary to know what constitutes an acceptable standard. This requires the articulation of technical knowledge and an understanding of the norms and values of the profession or institution, as the ideal can take various forms depending on the purpose of the evaluation (Jost, 1988, p. 5320). As with concepts of quality definitions of standards are often competing and poorly articulated. The difficulties of establishing performance criteria are also compounded by the diffusion of decision-making in the NHS.

Thirdly, an effective system must be able to measure current practice or services by applying the most suitable evaluation to circumstances, individuals and institutions. Such measures need to be reliable and valid and supported by rigorously conducted studies (Brook and Kosecoff, 1988). Currently, measurement studies are limited although the Department of Health has set in motion various schemes and projects to reduce deficiencies. But many measures of practice are far from being scientifically based, relying on anecdotal reports, consensus conferences and expert opinion. It is important to recognize that one of the pitfalls of quality assurance is the use of such measures as a substitute for the specification of a concept or failure to define the requisite standard.

Last, but not least, care must be taken that any quality assurance evaluation is capable of being translated into practice. This is likely to involve the development of training, education and incentive schemes to enable performance to be modified so that it conforms more closely to decided standards (Jost, 1988).

THE ROLE OF CONTRACT

In an effort to induce greater efficiency in the use of resources, the main focus of the reforms has been the creation of a 'provider or internal market'. The pivot of the new organization is the imposed use of contract as the vehicle which underpins the implementation of policy and provision of health services from April 1991. The contract mechanism is seen as having two main advantages. It separates the role and the responsibilities of purchasers of health care from that of providers. Just as importantly, by formally setting out criteria and targets for delivery, it is seen to provide a means of focusing both purchaser and provider attention on the quality of health care and supplying a catalyst for improvement.

These arrangements by which DHAs are to procure services are of especial interest to public lawyers. The purported intention is that accountability will be enhanced through the network of contractual obligations to be negotiated between purchasers and providers. This could provide an opportunity to develop health care which reflects community needs and preferences and for monitoring to be placed in a wider context which includes procedures for feedback from GPs and from patients themselves. However, in order to realize the potential of informed contracting the respective roles of medical professionals, managers and consumers need to be reappraised (Harvey, 1991). In particular the challenge for health authorities is to refrain from using any often inappropriate 'shopping analogies' and instead develop public management frameworks which are able to recognize and balance the disparate values and interests of the community as a whole.

Several implications arise out of the move to contract as a means of administering health care provision. In the first place and most importantly it has brought about a change in the role and functions of DHAs who have to some extent been required to minimize their activities in the day-to-day provision of health services and as already mentioned in the preceding chapter, evolve a consumer advocate role. DHAs now act as purchasing or commissioning agents, acquiring services on behalf of residents from a variety of providers: hospitals remaining under DHA management, self-governing NHS Trusts and the private sector.

In order to carry out this function one of the main tasks of DHAs has been to start to develop associations with other agencies concerned with health care in order to open communication channels about the availability of services, the pattern of their use and their evaluation. The resulting information, which is still very much in an embryonic stage, is expected to provide a basis for contractual arrangements about services. In the past DHAs have admittedly had very little genuine dialogue with the wider community and so the change requires a re-orientation of focus and culture and a difficult balancing of interests for DHA management (NHSME EL(90)).

Doubts must be raised about whether districts are equipped to manage the networks and associations necessary to produce a coherent organization. At present the structures and procedures which are imperative for the latter have been left very much to the discretion and initiative of district management and are nowhere detailed in the sequence of papers coming from the Department of Health and the NHS Management Executive. Consequently in carrying out exploratory discussions health authorities have forged some innovative mergers and unusual alliances. Whilst some health authorities are merging parts of their management structure with that of FHSAs or making joint appointments to some posts, others are forming purchasing consortia. Larger purchasing authorities can make economical use of buying power and expertise, save costs and eliminate duplication of information and are a logical progression particularly where ultimately there may be few or even no directly managed units as more service providers seek self-governing status (Moore, 1991).

However, only a few current alliances have undergone any public consultation or ministerial approval. Yet many of these purchasing partnerships are likely to be a precursor to more formal mergers. Thus the rebuilding of health authority boundaries and reshaping of organizational structures is being carried out in a largely *ad hoc* and unaccountable manner. There is a further risk, particularly as there are few formal structures for local representation and input, that larger, merged authorities might lose touch with the values and requirements of the local community (Ham, quoted in Moore, 1991). Although an analysis of these developments has been commissioned by the NHSME, in the interest of stability and cohesion some guidance and framework needs to be given rapidly to these developments to ensure that the above possibilities do not occur. Most of these changes are occurring not as a direct result of legislation, approved by Parliament, but as a result of administrative or management reorganization, the potential impact of which is enormous. Thus in terms of accountability DHA activities are very much an unchartered area and yet formally their constitutional position remains unchanged in that although they have separate legal identity as statutory corporations, they carry out their functions on behalf of the Secretary of State.

Secondly, contracting may have the unfortunate effect of cutting down choice of available services and of curtailing clinical freedom. As contracting structures become established and clinicians and GPs are expected to operate and refer within those patterns, exceptions are likely to have to be rigorously justified.

But, on a more positive note, the move to contract has a potential to make purchasing authorities far more explicit about their service priorities. Contracts have to be published. As contracting develops, content will become more detailed, specifying:

- the nature, level and quality of services required;
- the price, information and access necessary to monitor performance, and
- the available remedies if the terms of the contract fail to be met.

This should bring the allocation and rationing of health care into relief and result in an increase in public awareness.

A variety of contractual means are at the disposal of health authorities, each of which is subject to a different dispute resolution procedure. Genuine contracts, which give rise to traditional rights and obligations and which are governed by private law, will continue to be made between the public and private health care sectors; for example where a DHA or a funded general practice contracts with a private hospital, or a private purchaser such as an employer or insurance company contracts with an NHS hospital.

Alongside these conventional contracts a system of what could be termed 'public law contracts' operate. In English law there is no general concept of 'public law contract' as a means of governing commercial relationships between government or other public bodies and private firms, but in Europe the notion is accepted. In the USA concern that the contract mechanism was being used, in effect, to delegate public decision-making to private bodies has led to considerable debate about accountability in the 'contract state' (Harden and Lewis, 1986, p. 177). Although not uncontested (Jacob, 1991) the term seems to provide the best description of the development of new forms of formal agreements in the NHS. These developments have had the effect of making the boundaries of the concept of contract unclear.

Relations between units which remain district managed and their home authorities will be covered by management service agreements, 'arrangements structured as contracts but enforced through the normal management process'. In developing these arrangements the NHS Management Executive has stressed the importance of separating clearly the purchaser and provider roles within districts. The aim is to provide a broad framework within which the managed unit is free to operate but where it is also made clear when and how the DHA should be involved. As far as is practical district managed units are to be treated as self-sufficient providers, similar to NHS Trusts, the main difference relating only to factors concerned with financial and personnel management.

However, the requirement to evolve a framework to govern the separation of purchaser and provider roles and the relationship with managed units in effect amounts to setting up 'Chinese Walls' within authorities. This is likely to be difficult to maintain and has a potential to create further tensions which obscure rather than clarify the processes of accountability. Harden (1992) points out that the lack of any constitutional framework for the separation of interests between DHAs and managed units and the absence of a clearly defined role for DHAs independent of the Secretary of State could undermine the separation of provider and purchasing functions.

Arrangements with health service bodies outside the health authority management structure, namely NHS Trusts, are governed by a new kind of contract, the 'NHS contract' for which legislative provision was required and which specifically give rise to no contractual duties or liabilites at law. Such contracts are ultimately to be enforced not through the courts, but through arbitration powers exercised by the Secretary of State or a person appointed by him. It should be noted, however, that were a Trust to be in breach of an NHS contract it would be possible for the Secretary of State to apply for an order of mandamus or seek an injunction to enforce compliance. Although this is unlikely to occur, given the provision of alternative dispute-resolution procedures.

Guidance from the NHS management executive on resolving disputes states that all NHS contracts should be constructed so as to minimize the risk of dispute, but should include clauses for agreed arbitration if either party believes a contract has been broken. The parties to the contract should specify the arbitrator, who will usually be the Regional General Manager, but there appears to be no obstacle to the parties agreeing to private arbitration. They may also agree the terms on which arbitration may take place, including 'pendulum' arbitration where the arbitrator can only accept one or other of the parties position in full. This has the effect of forcing any compromises to be made before arguments are put to the arbitrator.

Arbitration clauses do not, however, alter the right of either party to use the formal dispute resolution procedure where informal procedures have failed.

Unusually, arbitration powers extend to pre-contractual negotiation if either party believes the other is making use of an unfair advantage. Where disputes arise over the terms of proposed contracts there is no agreed arbitration system. In that case, to obtain an impartial view of the proposed terms both parties are expected to seek the assistance of their Regional General Manager as conciliator. Once contract negotiations have begun neither party can withdraw without the permission of the other or the Secretary of State. This procedure is radically different from any in private law where regulation of this stage of contracting is unknown (Hughes, 1990, p. 432). The executive sees these arrangements, supported by a shared objective of securing effective health services as reducing the need for use of the formal dispute resolution process.

Where there is no apparent alternative to involving the formal procedure disputes will be referred to the Secretary of State. Cases where the Secretary of State decides to appoint an adjudicator to resolve a dispute are governed by The National Health Service Contracts (Dispute Resolution) Regulations (1991 SI 1991/725). The adjudicator may adopt a written procedure and may consult anyone whom he considers will assist him. The principles of natural justice are observed in the procedures. Each party is entitled to make representations, to see and comment on those made by the other party and to make observations on the results of any consultation. The adjudicator's decision has to be written and must be accompanied by reasons. Any determination of the Secretary of State, who has the power to vary the terms of the contract or to bring it to an end, is final and binding, although the above dispute-resolution powers are judicially reviewable.

Harden argues that although the formal framework and the requirement to give reasons has a potential to allow the development of principles which could clarify the policy framework for the contracting process, these are unlikely to emerge in practice. This is because the approach taken to dispute-resolution appears to be more akin to a managerial than a quasi-judicial process; formal resolution procedures are intended to be a last resort and the arbitration role of regional general managers is unlikely to be reviewable.

Furthermore, there is a discretion not to delegate formal disputes to an adjudicator in which case the Regulations do not apply.

Support is lent to this view by the fact that the Secretary of State is potentially an interested party rather than an independent arbiter in disputes because of his constitutional position in relation to health service authorities (Harden, 1992).

The effect of the above powers is that the actual degree of contractual freedom of purchasers and providers is ultimately determined centrally by executive decision, not by the market. The true nature of the contract mechanism in the health service therefore is not an undertaking of any commercial risk but merely another strategem for administrative planning. It is important that this is recognized because without the elements of risk and liability normally associated with contracting and competition, the growth between purchasers and providers of informal and therefore unaccountable 'orderings' to protect their mutual interests is likely to be sustained (Hughes, 1990; Hughes and Dingwall, 1990).

However, it is interesting to speculate whether NHS contracts might fall within the scope of the draft EC Services Directive which applies to contracts in writing, for pecuniary interest, between purchasers and suppliers where the 'purchaser' is a body governed by public law. The implications of the directive are that all such contracts have to be advertised in the *Official Journal of the EC* and are subject to a special regime governing the award of contracts. On the face of it a DHA intending to purchase services from an NHS Trust will have to comply with the directive. This could have the effect of opening up competition in the health care market and of rapidly undermining the mainly 'internal market' strategy of recent reforms (Harden, 1992).

Current contracts are generally on a 3-year rolling basis and formal review is assumed to take place yearly, either for renewal or up-dating and is expected to consider changes required in service specification due, for example, to any alterations in resources or priorities. Many of the contracts introduced in April 1991 were in block form which define a range of services for which there is an all-in set price. Although currently this has brought about little change from previous patterns of service, block form contracts are the starting point from which the government expect the process of contracting to develop and evolve. The importance and relevance of NHS contracts in this process will increase as and when more applications for NHS Trusts are approved.

Such processes may or may not improve health services for consumers, but a central question must be whether public accountability will be enhanced. The Department of Health has emphasized the importance of monitoring the quality of service provision. A critical issue in the contracting process is the setting of standards which meet the requirements of the purchaser and which the provider has an obligation to meet. In the event of a failure to meet standards the purchaser will be able to set in motion a review of the agreement. The Secretary of State has no powers to intervene on his own initiative nor does it appear that any third party has any right to refer a dispute for arbitration. An important question therefore is what rights, if any, might consumers have where there is a failure to meet agreed, publicly available standards?

Although the clear intention of the 1990 Act is to preclude the jurisdiction of the courts in relation to rights and liabilities that might otherwise arise between the parties, were NHS contracts subject to private law, it is arguable that this would not exclude in some circumstances an application for judicial review by some person or body with requisite standing. NHS Trusts and health authorities are public bodies within the National Health Service and it is feasible that the content of contractual agreements could give rise to a legitimate expectation of a defined quality or quantity of services for the consumer. Although the Secretary of State remains constitutionally, ultimately responsible for the general provision of health services under the 1977 Act, contracting makes more explicit the standards to be expected and achieved within resource limits. In the past applications for judicial review of failures to provide specific services have been unsuccessful because of a lack of any definition of what is actually to be provided (see Chapter 4). Where provision is articulated in a contract or set out as a standard in a charter, the courts might be prepared to lend support to the view that a legitimate expectation of a certain provision or quality of service has arisen. In these circumstances, some legal recognition would be given to the need for enhanced measures of public accountability for the increasing exercise of public power and delegated discretion through the medium of contract and quasi contract.

ACCOUNTABILITY FOR CLINICAL ACTIVITY

Jost points out that the first line of defence for assuring the quality of health care is through professional self-regulation which occurs through education and socialization processes, informal review by colleagues and more formal programmes for peer review such as medical audit (1988, p. 535). Self-regulation is of great value, but by itself is inadequate to ensure quality. As discussed below in relation to medical audit, the value of all means of self-regulation is contingent on the quality of the information provided and the use to which it is put.

Litigation has also played a part in quality of care, especially in relation to professional competence. If care deviates from the standard of adequate care established by the medical profession it may result in damages being awarded. Tort law defines and evaluates quality through lay analysis of the evidence of medical experts, who attempt to elucidate standards and describe how these have been conformed to or deviated from. However, negligence actions are fairly ineffective and ill-equipped to serve as a means of achieving overall quality. Firstly the selection of cases is very narrow – in the UK most victims never sue. Secondly judgements are long drawn out, often inconsistent and unpredictable. Thirdly there is no coherent or comprehensive feedback system to providers, purchasers or the public (Jost, 1988, pp. 572–6).

Much of the current activity to define and measure quality of health services is taking place against the traditional Donabedian trio of concepts which conflates and categorizes quality evaluation mechanisms as being concerned with inputs, process and outcome (Donabedian, 1966). Quality assurance task teams have been set up in health authorities, some jointly with others, whose primary responsibility is to develop measurable quality assurance criteria and standards for service specifications (see for example Bexley Health Authority et al., 1990). When many of these teams first met it was quickly established that little was known within the service about the task at hand and that patients, medical professionals and management potentially perceived structure, process and outcome from separate standpoints. A multi-faceted approach is therefore extremely important and health authorities are in the process of developing quality matrix in an attempt to take this into account.

The latest reorganization of the NHS places no reliance on increased funding for health services and instead concentrates on potential gains from a more efficient use of resources. Consequently a central theme is to find means to ensure that those concerned with the delivery of services not only make the best use of available resources but also become more accountable for that usage and for their own performance. To facilitate these concerns key proposals are an extension of the Resource Management Initiative (RMI) and the development of a system of 'medical audit' as part of routine clinical practice. Both processes have generally been welcomed and if properly deployed provide a potential to serve both the individual and collective elements of responsibility for effective and efficient use and delivery of health services.

THE RESOURCE MANAGEMENT INITIATIVE

In order for contracting to work effectively as the vehicle which underpins the provision of health services a comprehensive means of accounting for the utilization and costs of resources has to be established. The Resource Management Initiative (RMI) is the most recent method of management or clinical budgeting which aims to involve clinicians, whose decisions to a large extent determine the use of resources, more closely in the management and effective use of hospital services, through improved provision of information.

A few isolated and experimental schemes to involve clinicians in responsibility for the resources used in the care of their patients were tried in the 1970s and early 1980s. But the major impetus for the RMI came from the Report of the Griffiths Inquiry into NHS Management which explicitly challenged the view that clinical decisions about care should be isolated from any concern for costs and consequently recommended the development of:

> management budgets involving clinicians at unit level with an emphasis on management and not accountancy. The aim is to produce an unsophisticated system in which workload related budgets covering financial and manpower allocations and full overhead costs are closely related to workable service objectives and against which performance and progress can be measured.

> (Griffiths, 1983)

The Resource Management Initiative was introduced on an experimental basis at six sites in 1986. This has since been supplemented by quite a large number of local initiatives wanting to anticipate changes likely to come about when the demonstration projects had been concluded (Coombs and Cooper, 1990). When first established the programme was stated to be principally about altering the attitude of clinicians towards taking account of resource ultilization and encouraging closer team work amongst medical professionals and other managers in resource management. Before any decisions were to be taken about implementation in the rest of the health service a progress review of the six demonstration sites was to be published in October 1989. The review would be expected to demonstrate the efficacy of several concerns and claims for the RMI. The primary consideration was how to involve medical professionals in the management process so that they would be committed to taking responsibility for their use of resources and be better able to take decisions regarding service quality. The consequent systems evolved needed to show their feasibility in terms of running at an acceptable cost and their attraction for doctors by providing accurate and medically credible data of activity. The review would also have been expected to demonstrate the value of management information systems for nurses and departments like pathology, radiology and pharmacy and linked costing systems (Social Services Committee, 1989).

However, the events of the latest health service reform have overtaken a full analysis of the RMI (for a comprehensive text see Packwood *et al.*, 1991). In an attempt to bring clinicians even more surely within the framework of resource and financial accountability the reorganization has made changes to both the timetable for extension of resource management and its purpose. The focus of the RMI as presented in *Working for Patients* appears to be the provision of cost information:

. . . there is at present only a limited capacity to link information about the diagnosis of patients and the cost of treatment.

(*Working for Patients*, 1989, para. 2.14)

There is also an acceleration of the implementation of the initiative by a programme which was drawn up before a full review had been completed.

Concern has been expressed that the timetable for accelerated introduction is over-optimistic; not only has there been a lack of proper evaluation but staff training facilities are inadequate and running costs are likely to be substantial. In addition there is some evidence that the strength of opposition to involvement in resource management from the medical profession may have been underestimated (Pollitt, 1988).

As the Social Service Committee commented:

In sum from a very broadly based initiative where the changing of attitudes and the encouraging of team work in relation to resource management were central objectives, and where the

Joint Consultants Committee was to be involved in evaluation before further expansion of the RMI was agreed, the RMI is to become much more narrowly focused on costs and speeded up.
(Social Services Committee, 1989, para. 2.54)

The facilitation of resource management is a complex process which requires considerable investment in the development of financial and resource utilization information systems. This can only be justified if it can be demonstrated that increased benefits in the effectiveness and efficiency of the allocation and use of resources flow from the imposition of the RMI. The systems now being envisaged are a far cry from the 'unsophisticated system' recommended but never elucidated by Griffiths. Research is indicating that there are serious problems with the implementation of the RMI in terms of technical accounting difficulties, the availability of the necessary information technolgy and confusion about control and possession of the system (Coombs and Cooper, 1990; Packwood *et al.*, 1991).

Coombs and Cooper argue that information systems take on different forms depending on the balance of concerns represented during the process of development and identify two extreme perspectives of resource management, one that is clinically led, and the other that is financial management led. Emphasis on the latter can result in insufficient consideration being given to medical valuation of respective treatments. Furthermore it could result in a lack of attention being given to cost-dumping where savings in one area of health care are more than offset by additional costs in others. The main concern is that shifts in practice can be attempted through the development of information systems which fail to articulate that particular sorts of information are privileged and which serve to reinforce only particular and potent perspectives about what the NHS is, what its goals are and what its procedures should be (Coombs and Cooper, 1990, p. 9).

However, the potential gains for the NHS arising from the implementation and process of the RMI could be immense in relation to financial, professional and public accountability and could provide benefits for health service and organizational quality. Packwood and colleagues point out that although implementation may be slower than anticipated and as yet incomplete, much has been learned already. They conclude that there is a 'strong internal logic' to resource management as it enables services to be genuinely managed, promotes collaboration and combines 'authority and accountability for decisions about the allocation of resources, their management and planning and review of services into a coherent whole' (Packwood *et al.*, 1991, p. 157).

Thus properly considered and openly operated resource management can offer a chance for management, medical professionals and consumers to plan health services on a more rational basis by supplying evidence of use and needs and highlighting any requirement for change in the deployment of resources. It can therefore provide an opportunity for genuine local decision-making. Much depends on a theme that goes throughout this book; the gathering of necessary information, its interpretation and the use to which this is put. This does not necessarily mean emphasis on investment in the development of high technology data collection. Again, Packwood *et al.* point to many examples of benefits arising from resource management, not from the provision of sophisticated data, but from the improved capacity and means to agree and implement a strategy (Packwood *et al.*, 1991, p. 158).

Resource management could fail to reach its full potential if information gathering and use is restricted to cost effectiveness and excludes other equally important elements. RMI has as yet not had any impact on the relationship between providers and consumers although it may have resulted in some internal adjustments between different interest groups within the NHS (Packwood *et al.*, 1991, p. 161). Only if all those concerned with its exercise can see clearly and openly the benefits of the RMI, by it rendering visible what are now often tacit features of health care provision, will it be able to develop into a successful social resource for improving and assuring the quality of health services.

MEDICAL AUDIT

As part of the overall package of resource control a comprehensive system of medical audit is also being introduced. Medical audit is central to any programme to enhance overall quality of care and is described as a systematic and critical analysis of the quality of medical care, including the procedures used for diagnosis and treatment, the use of resources, and the resulting outcome and quality of life for the patient (Working Paper 6). The requirement to participate in audit has been included in consultant's contracts and GP terms of service and so there are no specific provisions for medical audit in the 1990 Act.

Forms of medical audit were already developing in some areas of clinical practice and much of what has been proposed by government has been welcomed by the medical profession as it reflects and builds on both national and local initiatives which have been encouraged and supported by the Royal Colleges and clinicians in general.

Because medical audit is regarded as requiring specialized knowledge of current medical practice and access to medical records the approach taken by government is based firmly on the principle of peer review. But as management have the task of monitoring the use of resources they have been given responsibility for ensuring that an effective system of audit is developed and might be expected to contribute to the constitution of audit schemes. The form of audit and the frequency of review are therefore a matter for negotiation between management and medical professionals locally. But as is the case with the RMI this might give rise to some tension about which group is entitled to lead the system.

It is intended that every doctor and medical team should participate in regular systematic audit, the results of medical audit in respect of individual patients and doctors remaining confidential at all times. However, general results are to be made available to local management in order to satisfy them that the appropriate remedial action has been taken where audit has revealed that problems are being experienced. If management are not satisfied that resources are being used to the best effect they can request the District Audit Advisory Committee to initiate an independent audit which may take the form of a peer review carried out by clinicians from outside the district or a joint professional and managerial appraisal of a particular service.

Each DHA has therefore had to establish an audit advisory committee, chaired by a senior clinician, whose membership includes representatives of major medical specialities, including a GP together with clinicians representing the District General Manager. The central role of the committee is to plan and monitor a comprehensive programme for audit which is expected to include ways of incorporating the perspectives of patients. Each committee will produce an annual forward plan which will specify the methods to be used and the frequency of audit for each clincial team and detail a rolling programme under which the treatment of particular conditions is to be reviewed collectively by the relevant clinicians. This is also expected to include longer term results involving collaboration with primary care.

The committee is also expected to produce an annual report on the previous year's activity which details procedures used and services covered together with any actual or recommended follow-up action where means of improving the quality or efficiency of care have been identified. It is suggested that relevant parts of both the forward plan and the annual report could be made available to other health authorities which are considering placing contracts within the district, but there is no mention of any further dissemination of audit information (Working Paper 6).

At regional level audit is supported once again through an Audit Advisory Committee whose remit is to work on behalf of district authorities and assist them in discharging their responsibilities for ensuring that suitable comprehensive audit covers all services. Members are drawn from the district committees to cover all speciality interests and each team will be expected to organize audit of the smaller specialities on a regional basis, arrange for clinicians to undertake any external review of particular problems in districts and advise and support the development of audit throughout the region. It would seem sensible for this committee to cover the needs of primary care audit as well, given the changing role of regional authorities in relation to FHSAs and the need to ensure coordination between the sectors.

As regards general practice the importance of medical audit or at least quality initiatives has been increasingly recognized by the profession and its supporting organizations. For example, schemes which inspect the practices in which new GPs are trained have been operating for some while. The system for general practice is envisaged as being based primarily on audit taking place within individual practices but these will be monitored by management. Each FHSA is required to establish a medical audit advisory group to 'lead, support and encourage peer review and self-audit by individual GPs and practices'. This group committee will parallel in many ways the work of the district medical advisory committee with which it will have cross-representation and will be accountable to the FHSA through the FHSA general manager. A smaller team from this group will take responsibility for surveying and reporting on internal audit procedures whilst the larger group will consider area-wide issues and report on action taken.

The provisions for medical audit have been widely welcomed by professional and consumer organizations, although there is some criticism. Taken at face value the purpose of medical audit is to evaluate the quality of care, but a closer look appears to suggest a lack of commitment on the part of government to develop adequate measures for actual monitoring and improvement of quality. This arises from a lack of clarity about the conception of audit with which government intends NHS management to operate, and the use to which medical audit may be put. McSweeney (1988) points out that audits are not just descriptions or judgements, the values underlying them not only influence responses to evaluation criteria but also influence awareness of both alternatives and priorities. As with resource management mechanisms there is a feeling that the primary concern is cost effectiveness which is evidenced by a confusion between medical audit and monitoring of value for money in NHS government literature. Both are legitimate and necessary processes but they are not the same thing. In negotiating and regulating contracts for the care of patients, health authorities need to take account of medical audit arrangements and results alongside those of other types of audit for overall quality and costs.

Furthermore, too narrow a focus may have been given to the factors which can affect the results of audit in relation to quality and outcomes in the acute sector. Whilst organizational arrangements for audit demand that differing needs of specialities working within hospital services and in primary care be taken into account and may because of those differences have to focus on variable aspects of quality, the differences between medical audit in hospital and in primary care have perhaps been over-emphasized. Although there may be practical difficulties in auditing general practice and episodes of ill-health may be more clearly defined in hospital care for some patients, care in hospital as well as primary care may continue over a number of years, involve different teams sharing medical records, and the quality of outcomes may be affected by environmental factors in all sectors of care (Working Paper 6, para. 5.2). It is important that the systems that develop do not do so independently of one another and are able to link information so that more complete evidence on the quality of the continuation of care between hospital and GPs and related services can be provided.

Like the RMI, medical audit requires a significant investment not only financially but in terms of clinicians' time and energies, as well as that of support staff, to ensure that the necessary information is available. At present information systems are no more than rudimentary, it takes long consideration and time to develop and refine measures into useful medical and management tools. Good examples of audit need to be documented, evaluated and then disseminated so that others can learn and build on proven methods and utilize findings. And yet the government appears to have underestimated the scale of the task and costs. The amount of money made available from the central fund established for the purpose has been described as 'woefully inadequate' (Social Services Committee, 1989). Additionally medical audit should not preferably be restricted to clinicians. To do this could result in a lack of understanding of how care is integrated and lead to an inaccurate assessment of quality standards. It is quite possible for outcomes to be distorted or misinterpreted by a failure to include activity other than that of clinicians. Quality standards need to be set and audit carried out on the basis of the whole health care team so that a clear picture can be obtained. Provision of quality care is in fact a spiral learning process which continually links needs and care (Mallet, 1991, pp. 24–5).

As regards audit of general practice there is a suspicion that the aims of these procedures is to investigate variations in GP referral patterns which may then be used to enforce budgetary limits by discouraging referrals and assist the FHSA in developing the system of indicative budgeting and 'referral packages' not dissimilar to those now being developed for drugs use. However, this is unlikely. Referrals are a poor indication of the quality of general practice and any curtailment would cause considerable difficulties with clinical autonomy (Hughes, 1991, p. 101). There are no indications of what action is to be taken in cases where unacceptable standards are found in general practice. Neither is it clear whether the proposals relate to audit of the practice, for example its facilities and appointment procedures, or to an audit of clinical outcomes, or both.

The various means of quality assurance undoubtedly supplement and complement one another. But for several reasons doubt persists that the systems which are now being promoted are adequate to provide true review and monitoring of quality.

In the first place there is an overall preoccupation with the quantification of results. Information on outcomes needs to be considered alongside data on activity levels, cost and length of stay to demonstrate that improvements are real and that increased activity or quantity is not at the expense of quality. Such a development might result in increased re-admission and complication rates.

Secondly, there is as yet an inability to generate accurate information. Much of that which is available is still of questionable accuracy and hence marginal utility. In effect information systems are as yet at no more than the 'model T' stage (McClure, 1988). Further, some programmes being developed cannot be fully relied on to produce a true quality evaluation because they too easily serve other purposes that are concurrent and sometimes compete with quality evaluation functions.

Thirdly, quality assurance systems operate in some sectors of health care less effectively than others as schemes are not easily transferable and need to be tailored to context. For example some systems may deal well with activity in the acute sector but may have little application to the long-term care of those who are mentally handicapped, elderly or chronically ill. The lesson is that quality assurance schemes themselves need to be seriously and carefully evaluated before being implemented.

In the USA there is a much deeper commitment to reducing the above deficiencies. The federal government funds research to define quality and examine quality evaluation tools. Recently support has been provided for an examination of the relationship between variations in practice and quality, and between quality of care and health outcomes in several areas of clinical activity. In addition, Peer Review Organizations (PRO) provide a primary means of obtaining evaluative information on health care quality as they receive and generate a vast quantity of data. Although PRO regulations limit public release of information they do permit disclosure of quality data regarding health care institutions. Furthermore, a majority of states have now passed legislation to compel release of information collected by providers (Jost, 1988).

CONSULTANT CONTRACTS

Allied with increased accountability of the medical profession for the resources they use and the extension of the RMI and medical audit has been the introduction of new style consultant contracts. District management now has a clearer role in specifying the duties and responsibilities of consultants which places them in a better position to monitor performance against contractual obligations. Previously, with the exception of consultants working in Teaching Districts or Special Health Authorities, contracts were held by RHAs which caused 'some confusion about the nature of a consultants accountability to local management and the DHA'. To improve accountability processes, DHAs have been appointed to act as managing agents for regional authorities to work out acceptable arrangements for consultant duties. This change, like that of medical audit, did not require any new legislative provisions as it was consistent with the existing terms of consultant contracts.

As part of the same process every consultant has had to agree a more detailed job description with local management. These set out the main duties and responsibilities of the post including details of clinical, teaching and administrative elements, a work programme detailing each day's main duties and their location, participation in medical audit, out of hours commitments and budgeting and management obligations. Job descriptions are renewable annually to provide an opportunity for consultants and management to discuss any changes needed to meet changing circumstances or service priorities, but government expects that amendments will generally be minimal and infrequent. Although NHS Trusts employ their own consultants they are subject to the new appointment procedures and distinction award system.

Changes have also been made to procedures for the appointment of consultants. Previously there was no provision for district management to take any formal part in this process. Appointments are recommended by the Advisory Appointments Committees (ACC) whose membership is predominantly professional and whose primary consideration is professional suitability. RHA and DHA officers could previously only attend ACC meetings at the invitation of the committee and then were not allowed to sit as members. The Appointment of Consultant Regulations have now been amended to enable District General Managers and the Chief Executive of NHS Trusts to be full members of ACCs in order that a consultant's willingness and ability to meet the requirements of the post for the management of resources and development of services can be examined. Similar trends can be seen in the changes made to the system of distinction awards which are now to take account of resource and service development achievements as well as clinical skills.

In conclusion, when resources are limited it is important and realistic to ensure that there are effective accountability processes for clinical activity, but it is equally important that these should not focus exclusively on the containment of costs to the detriment of quality and other fundamental social values. We must also be watchful that the burden of expenditure is not merely shifted onto other agencies through various manipulative tactics. Monitoring systems need to be opened up to encourage co-operation and to ensure that public expenditure as a whole is used as effectively and efficiently as possible for publicly established purposes. The Audit Commission could play an enhanced role in this.

THE ROLE OF THE AUDIT COMMISSION

To assist the aim of better value for money in the provision of health care the government has made changes in the arrangements for audit of the accounts of health authorities. Section 20 of the 1990 Act has amended Pt III of the 1982 Local Government Finance Act (LGFA) and made provision for external statutory audit of all NHS bodies, including NHS Trusts and fund-holding general practices, by the transference of responsibility from the Department of Health to the Audit Commission. This does not affect the separate roles of the Comptroller and Auditor General and the National Audit Office which remain unaltered. The Comptroller and Auditor General will continue to report to Parliament on the use of voted funds and NHS resources investigated by the National Audit Office and to certify the aggregated accounts of the NHS, drawing on audits of the Commission.

Under the LGFA 1982 the Audit Commission, now renamed the Audit Commission for Local Authorities and the National Health Service in England and Wales, has two distinct responsibilities relating to the estimation of value for money in the services to which the provisions apply. Firstly S26(1), which applies in full to the Commission's new role in the NHS, requires the Commission to undertake or promote studies into the economy, efficiency and effectiveness in the provision of services. Secondly, S27(1) requires that the Commission reports on the impact of the operation of statutes, directions and guidance on the economy, efficiency and effectiveness in the provision of services or on financial management. This latter provision was initially excluded from arrangements for the NHS, ostensibly because of the difference between accountability arrangements for local authorities and the NHS.

Accountability for the provision of health services was seen as being greater and clearer than that of local services. Health authorities are accountable to the NHS Management Executive which has responsibility for the impact of health policy. The Management Executive is in turn responsible to the Policy Board, chaired by the Secretary of State, who is accountable to Parliament for policy and management of the NHS. However, after some debate the Commission's hand was strengthened; by Para 19, Schedule 4 of the 1990 Act the Audit Commission may take full account of the implementation of statutes, directions and guidance, subject to its not questioning the policy objectives of the Secretary of State for Health. The Parliamentary Under-Secretary of State for the Department of Social Security explained that this latter provision reflected professional practice audit which reported on regularity and value for money in the implementation of policy rather than dispute underlying objectives (*Hansard* H.L. Vol. 520, col. 265). This of course assumes that a clear division between policy and implementation is possible.

The foregoing arrangements have been widely welcomed as a real and valuable form of external reporting on health care provision. The independence of the Audit Commission from central and local government and the NHS is underpinned by the financial structure within which it operates, as audited bodies pay for their own audits. The 15–20 Commission members are appointed by the Secretaries of State for the Environment, Health and Wales, after consultation with local and health authority associations and others, and are drawn from local government, the NHS trade unions, the accounting profession and private industry. In addition to financial audit the Audit Commission has already gained substantial experience in publishing performance indicators and identifying good practice in local authority services, including those related to health such as care of the elderly and care of those with mental handicap. In a memorandum to the Social Services Select Committee the Audit Commission has stated that it expects to adopt a similar approach to health care provision (Memorandum from the Audit Commission R151 HC 1988–89 214-IV).

The Commission has adopted straightforward definitions of economy, efficiency and effectiveness:

● Economy is the need to minimize the cost of inputs.
● Efficiency is the process of maximizing the productivity of those inputs.
● Effectiveness is the extent to which the output generated meets the objectives set for the service or the needs of those to whom it is delivered. Most effectiveness measures can also be seen as measures of quality of service. (The Audit Commission, 1991, p. 8).

The balance of emphasis given to 'economy, efficiency and effectiveness' depends on the kind of study undertaken or the main emphasis may be on management process which the Commission sees as encompassing all three.

The Commission has been criticized mainly on two counts. Firstly, that the regulatory role played by auditors can constrain local flexibility and political choice; and secondly, that there has been too little emphasis on effectiveness in the reports issued. The commission does not accept either of these claims, pointing out that it works within a well-established legislative framework and there is no persuasive evidence, including that from outside studies, that the effectiveness remit of auditors has been underplayed.

In the next few years the Audit Commission (1991, pp. 24–6) has stated that it is to focus on several concerns that have emerged as needing priority action in the public sector. These are:

- *Shifting the focus from inputs to outputs.* This is intended eventually to produce a number of additional measures of service quality.
- *Assessment of consumer views.* For example, material has been published on assessing satisfaction with day surgery, which includes a questionnaire for use by health authorities to assess their own performance.
- *Monitoring.* The development of the purchaser/provider split has made it essential that contracts are monitored effectively to ensure quality of services and value for money are obtained. This requires the development of measures of need, quality assurance, and new management skills. Studies of the role of the purchaser in the NHS are now underway and will focus on these areas.
- *Improvement of consumer input.* The Commission recognizes that there must be mechanisms for the inclusion of consumer views into service planning that is consistent with available resources and has stated that this is an area in which more work needs to be done.
- *Development of new management skills.* A consistent theme emerging from work done so far in the NHS is that managers lack the skills to manage change, and the Commission believes it has a facilitating role to play here by producing forward-looking reports.
- *Coordinating services.* Health policy initiatives can affect more than one agency or cut across departments and units, but there is often a lack of co-ordination between those concerned. Multi-agency and intra-agency audits are being planned to help improve co-operation.
- *Joint-working with professional audit.* In the NHS there is a developing body of medical audit work, the Health Advisory Service and others promoting quality standards and good practice. The Commission's distinctive contribution to these is seen as bringing an independent perspective, but care should also be

taken to avoid duplication and ensure co-operation. Liaison arrangements with the National Audit Office are already in place but links need to be developed with other bodies.

Taken together the new responsibilities of the Audit Commission, the extension of the RMI and the introduction of medical audit seem to indicate a clear intention by the government to speed up the development of formal performance measurement. The Select Committee pointed out the importance of not duplicating work and facilitating co-operation between all those concerned in all forms of audit, both external and internal with a view to establishing single sets of indicators, including suitable means of assessing outcomes that can be used by health bodies for management purposes and will also form a basis for objective value for money analysis by the Audit Commission (Social Services Committee, 1989, para. 3.8–3.12).

The Audit Commission appears to be taking this on board in setting priorities for its future approach. This may go some way to alleviating the difficulties that all audit devices display – namely their tendency to over-simplify and quantify issues and, just as importantly, their use in isolation from other performance indicators. Together these factors may give the impression of a breadth of information which exceeds reality (McSweeney, 1988, p. 28).

CONCLUSION

This chapter has dealt primarily with the implementation of health policy and the development of evaluative mechanisms. Though of fundamental importance for accountability these latter measures are only recently coming to receive the attention they deserve within the NHS. The different, basic concepts of quality need different procedures to ensure that they are facilitated. Of prime importance in this development of standards and performance criteria is the avoidance of the implementation of underfunded, second-rate quality assurance schemes. As Brook and Kosecoff (1988) argue, this could result in neither cost savings nor improvements in overall health status and could, in the long term, possibly generate more harm than good. The central argument is that law can play an important part in guiding providers and purchasers in the need to balance financial and quality concerns by providing the framework in which the different elements of quality can be taken into account, standards can be set and evaluative systems can be designed and applied.

Currently doubts must be raised about the use to which the contract mechanism, resource management and medical audit are to be put and the adequacy of the information systems being introduced. Concern must also be expressed about the lack of procedures for the dissemination of resultant information on a more widespread scale. It is important that health policy is constrained from putting too great an emphasis on cost containment at the expense of quality and other social values. There is a need to establish measures which encourage the collection and responsible release of information on health care quality so that policy choices are made on a sounder basis and an improved knowledge of potential difficulties. This in turn would help ensure more effective and efficient public expenditure.

4

PATIENTS AND PERSEVERANCE: GRIEVANCES AND RESOLUTION

GRIEVANCE REDRESS AND ACCOUNTABILITY IN THE NHS

This chapter deals with the fourth law-job, the resolution of disputes. It concentrates on grievances which might have a potential bearing on policy decisions rather than those concerned with individual mistakes of medical practice. The latter, which are usually resolved through private law procedures for the tort of medical negligence, have become a frequent topic of debate in recent years and are covered extensively in other literature.

But it is worthwhile noting at this point that current procedures for resolving medical negligence claims are both lengthy and cumbersome and can have a profound impact on health authority budgets. Since 1 January 1990 health authorities have been wholly responsible for negligence claims, resulting in an expenditure of £45 million by the NHS in that year. Consequently certain measures have recently been taken to reduce costs. Under the Court and Legal Services Act 1990 all personal claims under £50 000 will now normally be dealt with in the County Court, although a provision exists for more complicated cases to be transferred to the High Court even if below this financial limit. New rules also require earlier disclosure of medical records and improved pre-trial exchange of factual materials and witness statements in an attempt to clarify issues, reduce delays and encourage settlement.

The most recent proposal is for a panel of three, comprising two doctors, one nominated by each party, and a lawyer experienced in medical negligence claims to provide a voluntary arbitration scheme. The scheme would come within the general framework of the Arbitration Acts and is intended to supplement, not replace present arrangements (Arbitration for Medical Negligence; Department of Health, 1991). The proposals can be criticized on several counts. The take-up rate of the scheme may not be high enough to justify it being set up. It is unlikely that there will be sufficient cases of a simple enough nature which can be dealt with without a provision for oral evidence, which present proposals exclude. Less complex claims are already usually settled out of court and the more complicated cases may be unsuitable for a decision based only on written submissions and medical records. In addition, it is currently intended that the costs of the scheme should fall on the parties involved, as they do under the normal rules of arbitration. But, even though there may be some savings in terms of legal fees, doubts must be expressed as to whether these will adequately cover the additional costs which the scheme will entail. Comments on the arbitration scheme were submitted by many interested groups at the invitation of the Department of Health and it remains to be seen whether it is established as proposed.

The theme throughout this book is that there is a need to take a closer look at accountability processes and public input into NHS policy. From the point of view of a public lawyer, complaints and their handling are a fundamental aspect of accountability; part of a belief that in a democratic system there must be an opportunity for the public to air and redress their grievances. A lack of effective avenues for complaints resolution is in itself an injustice. It has already been argued that in the modern state the possibility of participating in decision-making through the usual democratic channels has been undermined. Complaints processing may help to alleviate this tendency by allowing decisions to be challenged and investigated, which can then in turn provide a wider base of information for decision-making. Complaints procedures may therefore attain a degree of indirect consumer involvement in policy processes as well as contribute to a reputation for fair dealing, and so help legitimize health policy.

The proper handling of complaints aids a questioning process and the setting up of a dialogue between consumers and the institution complained against. When handled effectively this can be an important factor in monitoring the quality of day-to-day health care provision and indicate where resource responsibilities lie. By locating responsibility and bringing to light gaps in management systems, complaints procedures can contribute to management information and assist in the pursuit of efficiency.

However, the relationship between grievance redress and the managerial enterprise is far from straightforward. The mere provision of complaints procedures is not necessarily any indication that they work effectively. Nor can a lack of complaints or patient satisfaction be taken to be an indication of a good quality service. Even though patients may be treated sympathetically this can be the result of a benign web of informal grievance handling. Underlying this there may be a whole submerged body of complaints which the administrative or management culture has helped to suppress. Complaints processes thus possess a potential to individualize and to channel grievances into an acceptable forum, instead of allowing real or underlying issues such as a reduction in resources or a change in policy to be confronted. In such a way attention may be diverted from resource decisions to issues of maladministration.

But this need not be the case, as long as attention is paid to this tendency through the development of well-publicized and accessible complaints procedures and a positive culture of rights for consumers is encouraged. In this way it is possible to establish grievance procedures as a supplement to other political processes. By indicating the problem of scarce resources or their inefficient use concerns are brought into the political arena (Seneviratne, 1991).

In recent years there has been increased interest in the redress of grievances which has been strongly influenced by consumer movements. The American attitude is clearly expressed by Rosenblum;

> No set of guidelines, rules or principles can assure individual gratification over policy decisions; but the allocation of adequate skills, resources and procedures to the handling of citizen complaints and grievances can assure accountable responsive government sensitive to the needs and concerns of the ordinary American and entitled to his confidence and support.
>
> (Rosenblum, 1974)

In general there is a discernible change in the climate and culture of complaining, evidenced by an increasing number of available mechnanisms for reviewing action and by attempts on the part of some organizations to reduce the psychological and cultural barriers which have acted as a significant deterrent in the past. But it is also important that measures which aim to prevent disputes arising in the first place such as consultation, monitoring and other good practice measures are neither forgotten nor remain under-developed.

Within the NHS, credibility rests partly on patients being confident that their grievances will be dealt with in an equitable and just, as well as sympathetic manner. In examining the process of grievance resolution it is important to look at both internal procedures and external agencies such as the courts and the Health Service Commissioner to evaluate the significance of the role they play. As yet there is little empirical evidence about the way procedures are interpreted and incorporated into the work of personnel in the various health authorities. But that which is being done indicates there are many different approaches and practices in the way health authorities and FHSAs respond to consumer complaints (Longley, 1992).

Procedures for handling complaints about the provision of services in the NHS fall into three main categories according to the type of grievance and the identity of the party against whom the complaint is made. These variations reflect the different structural relationships which exist between the providers of services: health authorities, hospitals, GPs and family health service authorities.

HOSPITAL COMPLAINTS

Formal complaints about hospital services which do not involve the exercise of clinical judgement are referred to the relevant DHA under the terms of Health Circular 88(37) which set out directions issued by the Secretary of State under Section 1 of the Hospital Complaints Procedure Act 1985. Each health authority must designate a senior officer for each hospital or group of hospital units for which it is responsible to deal with complaints. Nominally this is usually the unit general manager but the actual job of processing complaints is dealt with by a member of their staff. Each district headquarters also has an officer designated to coordinate and deal with complaints on behalf of the District General Manager.

Complaints which concern the exercise of clinical judgement by hospital medical staff are dealt with under procedures set out in HC(81)5 and may be made either to the consultant concerned or directly to the DHA. In either case at this initial stage it is the responsibility of the consultant to look at the clinical aspects of the grievance and inform the district or unit manager of any significant risk of legal action or non-clinical aspects. If the complainant is dissatisfied with the consultant's reply, the complaint can be referred in writing to the Regional Medical Officer (RMO) who will then try to resolve it. If there is still no resolution the RMO has a discretion to arrange for a second opinion to be given by means of an Independent Professional Review (IPR) by two independent consultants. On completion of such a review it is the responsibility of the district or unit manager to inform the complainant of the result and any appropriate action taken. Complaints about clinical judgement do not come within the jurisdiction of the Health Service Commissioner (HSC) but the exercise of the discretion of the RMO whether to refer the complaint for independent review can be investigated by the HSC.

The occupational status of the designated officer in the units and at district headquarters varies between health authorities and it is important to note that complaints processing is only one aspect of their overall job. From the research conducted so far it appears that this factor may be having an effect on the way in which complaints are actually dealt with, the time and emphasis given to grievances and the use of complaints as an aspect of quality control (Longley, 1992). The guidelines themselves allow a great deal of discretion in both the processing and monitoring of complaints and there is consequently a wide variation in the organization and operation of procedures.

Health authorities are under a duty to monitor arrangements for grievance resolution in order to identify trends and direct that appropriate action is taken. Summaries of complaints have to be provided at quarterly intervals for consideration by either the authority itself, a committee of the authority or specified authority members. Again, although the Department of Health is now encouraging all health authorities to monitor complaints more systematically progress is spasmodic and monitoring is more generally taken to refer to the progress made with individual complaints rather than consideration of overall organizational deficiencies. Complaints about hospital services generally fall into three categories:

● environmental and support services, which cover 'hotel' services and other facilities;
● care, which covers clinical and non-clinical aspects from medical, paramedical and non-medical staff, and
● organization, which covers matters of general administration including the handling of complaints.

During the current reorganization grievance resolution has tended to take a back seat in some health authorities with the result that there are instances of failures to pick up delays and inefficiencies and a shelving of monitoring procedures. Paradoxically, the changes in NHS organization are in some instances benefiting complaints procedures. The focus on consumerism has led to increased enthusiasm amongst various groups to expand and develop monitoring of consumer views, including complaint patterns and trends, for use in the wider purchasing forums that are being created.

An example of good, systematic monitoring can be given from a health authority recently the subject of research where there had been an increase in complaints, over all three categories of grievances, which related either directly or indirectly to the provision of midwifery services. Policy on domiciliary midwives had been changed and dissatisfaction with the new practice showed up in various forms in a number of grievances. As a result of further investigation and effective monitoring by a quality control team the new policy was adjusted to take account of patient grievances and complaints were reduced. For trends such as this to be spotted much depends on the quality and efficiency of monitoring processes themselves. In a significant number of health authorities complaints monitoring mechanisms are as yet either underdeveloped or are only just in the process of becoming established.

The Association of Community Health Councils for England and Wales, whose members play a significant role in assisting complainants to bring their grievances to the attention of health authorities, have laid down five, overlapping criteria for successful complaints-handling (1990). These are visibility, accessibility, impartiality and fairness, and effectiveness and speed. To these could be added accountability and quality improvement. Complaints mechanisms must be publicized and grievances must be able to be made with a minimum of difficulty. Most health authorities have gone some way to ensuring this by the production of leaflets, notices and admission booklets which give information about how to complain and to whom. However, the quality and availability of these varies. It cannot be said that a positive culture of a right to complain has yet been established, and there has been some opposition to such publicity from clinicians who fear that spurious grievances might increase. Only a small number of health authorities provide any special leaflet or training for staff on how to handle complaints or where to refer patients so that matters can be dealt with appropriately.

Most complaints are written, but oral complaints are accepted and registered by hospitals and health authorities, and a record of the grievance has to be made by the complaints officer, which the complainant is then asked to sign. Guidance states that a refusal to sign should not delay the process of investigation. But there is a danger that oral complaints received by telephone may not be followed through as systematically as written ones. Memos of telephone complaints are often brief and may necessitate a later request for a written explanation, or increasingly a face-to-face interview. Hospitals and units are in general more frequently inviting patients to meet with staff complained against to discuss their grievances on an informal basis. This is good practice which often proves beneficial to the patient and all concerned as it can relieve misunderstanding and supply the explanation which the complainant seeks. But some caution must be expressed here. Such 'trouble shooting' practices are not preventive channelling in the law-job sense and may not bring to the attention of decision-makers what lies at the bottom of the complaint. It is important, therefore, that a record is kept of meetings between patients and staff, followed by a report which details the essence of the discussion which can then be fed into the monitoring process.

The Department of Health and health authorities are concerned about delay in grievance redress. Most authorities acknowledge the receipt of complaints quickly and guidance suggests a resolution time of a maximum of three weeks. A significant number of complaints fail to meet this target, particularly where the complaint involves more than one aspect. In that situation the time taken to respond increases because of the number of personnel who have to produce a report. Some complaints are ongoing for a number of weeks or months, so that it is of prime importance that complainants are kept abreast of progress, or the lack of it.

Any assessment of complaint handling must look carefully at the actual process of investigation so that any blockages or unfair practices might be spotted. By comparison of different authority procedures it should be possible to identify ways of reducing delay or partiality. Access to health records should help alleviate the difficulties faced by some complainants, especially those concerning clinical judgement. However, a frequent problem is likely to be the quality of records themselves for these purposes. This is something about which the Health Service Commissioner has commented on several occasions. Record keeping is of paramount importance in all aspects of clinical and management processes as they can help contribute to an equalization of the balance of power and openness of the organization.

Good grievance-handling practice means that complainants must receive a full explanation of what went wrong and an apology where appropriate. Information should include details of how to refer a grievance to an appropriate higher authority such as the Regional Medical Officer or the Health Service Commissioner if no satisfaction has been obtained at ground level, of any action taken to prevent a recurrence of the complaint. It is at this point where effective monitoring processes come into their own by providing feedback for the operation of the organization. Some health authorities and Trusts are establishing committees which regularly examine complaints files for the purpose of identifying specific areas for possible improvement.

On the whole hospitals and health authorities are becoming more aware of the necessity to handle complaints effectively. But there is still much to be done in terms of impartiality, accountability and the use of complaints as a factor in setting standards. More consideration needs to be given to the appointment of full-time complaints officers to act as a focal point for individual resolution and take responsibility for monitoring processes. Effective coordination of grievance handling is likely to become even more essential as DHAs seek to establish themselves as purchasers of quality services.

FAMILY HEALTH SERVICES AUTHORITIES

Complaints about family practitioners are dealt with by the relevant FHSA with whom GPs are contracted to provide services. FHSAs were issued with new, very extensive guidelines from the Department of Health in April 1990, following changes made by the National Health Service (Service Committees and Tribunal) Amendment Regulations 1990. These provisions coincided with the introduction of the new GP contract. These guidelines, in contrast to those issued to health authorities, are very detailed and comprehensive and at first sight appear to leave little discretion to complaints officers for their operation.

Each FHSA has to appoint an officer whose sole job, in contrast to health authorities, is to deal with procedures relating to complaints. Depending on the nature of the complaint grievances may be dealt with either by an informal or formal procedure. In the informal procedure a lay conciliator is appointed by the FHSA to try to resolve the complaint. FHSAs can only formally investigate alleged breaches of terms of service which may include clinical judgement or other matters.

The complaint must be made within 13 weeks of the cause of action and is referred to a medical service committee for investigation. A report is then made to the FHSA for a decision. Service committees may only consider specific allegations and incidents which might show a breach of contract. They are not allowed to take account of a history of poor practice. A medical service committee consists of three lay and three professional members in addition to the chairperson, but members receive little or no training and have to gain experience on the job. The effectiveness of committees varies widely, depending partly on the questioning skill and confidence of the members and partly on that of the chair (ACHCEW, 1990).

The Health Service Commissioner (HSC) has no jurisdiction to investigate the actions of GPs in connection with services provided under contract with FHSAs or action taken by FHSAs under the formal complaints procedure described above, but an appeal by either party does lie to the Secretary of State for Health. Delays to medical service committee hearings and appeals to the Minister are often protracted, benefiting neither the complainant nor the practitioner.

What is most striking is the difference in practice and interpretation of each FHSA within quite stringent regulations and guidelines. Any evaluation of complaints procedures needs to examine these differences in depth. Although there is currently no requirement to monitor trends in GP complaints this may alter as requirements for FHSAs to oversee GP practices and audit takes hold. Some 'informal' informal practices may be emerging. This may be because FHSAs are meant only to investigate complaints which indicate a breach of a GP's terms of service, but patients are more generally concerned with grievances that may not amount to a breach but which relate more to the quality of care and attitude of the GP. Complaints officers may see the resolution of such complaints as part of their job and steadily build up 'unofficial' ways of dealing with certain kinds of complaints with the district's contracted GPs. This practice can reduce the number of complaints that proceed to informal resolution by the lay conciliator and those that go for formal consideration by a Medical Service Committee. But here too there is a potential danger, mentioned before, that such practices may result in complaints being resolved to patient and practitioner satisfaction but may prevent important issues of collective interest coming to the fore.

THE HEALTH SERVICE COMMISSIONER

The post of HSC was created by the National Health Service Reorganization Act 1973 (see now the National Health Service Act 1977, Part V) and provides a service which is free to the complainant, is independent of the NHS and government and is accountable to Parliament. He reports three times a year to the Secretaries of State for Health with a selection of cases on which full investigations have been completed and produces an annual report, all of which are laid before Parliament.

The HSC can investigate complaints that an NHS body has not provided a service which it has a duty to provide, or failed in the provision of a service which is provided, or complaints about maladministration connected with action taken by or on behalf of an NHS authority. Some of the main areas investigated by the HSC over recent years include the care of the mentally handicapped, the registration and supervision of private nursing homes, the operation of the clinical complaints procedure and the behaviour of the FHSAs (HSC Annual Reports, 1986–91). Although instructed not to investigate action where an aggrieved person has a right of appeal to an administrative tribunal or court of law, in appropriate cases this requirement can be waived. To carry out thorough investigations the Health Commissioner can require health authorities to produce all relevant documents.

Complainants must show that they have suffered injustice or hardship as a result of the failure in service or from maladministration. Maladministration covers such matters as not following proper procedures or agreed policies, failing to have proper procedures, giving wrong information or inadequate explanations of care, or not dealing promptly or thoroughly with the original complaint.

The HSC cannot investigate a complaint about services provided by family doctors, dentists, opticians and pharmacists or action taken by an FHSA under the formal complaints procedure, namely the operation of service committees. And yet oddly he can investigate other aspects of the work of FHSAs such as the closure of surgeries and the removal of patients from a doctor's list.

Complaints about personnel matters such as staff appointments, pay, pensions and discipline, commercial and contractual dealings by health authorities and NHS Trusts are also outside the HSC jurisdiction.

However, the most important matter excluded from investigation are complaints, which in the HSC's opinion, concern solely the exercise of clinical judgement in the provision of diagnosis, care or treatment. What is or is not a matter of clinical judgement is sometimes difficult to discern and it is often argued that the jurisdiction of the HSC should be expanded to cover clinical judgement and complaints about family practitioners.

Complaints must generally be made within 1 year of the matter coming to the notice of the complainant. There is direct access to the HSC as long as the complaint has been made in the first instance to the health authority concerned and they have been given an adequate opportunity to investigate and explain it. One exception to this is when a complaint has been made by a member of staff or a hospital or health authority on behalf of a patient who is unable to complain for himself. In this case before accepting the complaint the HSC has to be satisfied that there is no one more appropriate. CHCs cannot make complaints about services to the HSC themselves, but they may assist or write on a complainant's behalf. In some circumstances health authorities may ask the HSC to investigate a complaint referred to them which they feel unable to resolve. However, this occurs rarely and requires a resolution of the members of the relevant authority.

Besides health authorities, NHS Trusts are also subject to HSC investigation. Although the HSC has yet to comment on the exclusion of contractual matters which are of increasing significance under recent NHS arrangements, concern has been expressed about the effect on complaints of the independence of Trusts. Trusts are directly accountable to the Secretary of State through the NHSME, although there are plans for RHAs to monitor performance of Trusts as agents of the Secretary of State. Although complaints against NHS Trusts are subject to the Hospital Complaints Procedure Act 1985 some Trusts have expressed the view that DHAs should have no interest in the handling of Trust complaints. The Deputy Commissioner has taken the view that monitoring of complaints is a feature of quality assurance and contract negotiation and therefore an essential concern for district authorities. It is important that grievances do not fall through any gap between the respective responsibilities of the two bodies. The position of Trust accountability for complaint handling will hopefully be clarified when guidelines are issued to the effect that district authorities should seek to monitor complaints and their handling through the insertion of appropriate clauses and terms in NHS contracts for the provision of services.

The exclusion of matters of clinical judgement has been a subject of long-standing controversy. By far the largest number of complaints rejected by the HSC concern clinical complaints. Added to these are those rejected because they clearly involve issues of medical negligence for which a legal remedy is available. As already indicated part of this excluded area is covered by the clinical complaints procedure adopted in 1981 which provide for an independent professional review (IPR) of clinical complaints by two consultants. The decision whether or not there should be an IPR is a discretionary one, taken by the regional medical officer (RMO). Consequently the HSC is empowered to investigate complaints about maladministration of the RMO, or the health authority concerned in the procedures leading up to or following the decision on an IPR. He can also consider the actions of the independent consultants who conduct the IPR.

It is understandable that reservations should be entertained about ombudsmen second-guessing the judgement of medical professionals. Although the IPR has been quite effective in identifying defects in procedures associated with the cause of complaint, each year the HSC has included in his reports cases illustrating problems which have arisen with the process. The HSC has consistently recognized that clinical judgement is not the sole prerogative of clinicians. There are occasions when the actions of nurses, midwives and other professionals also involve to some degree the exercise of clinical judgement and are therefore outside HSC jurisdiction. In those cases traditionally there has been no complaints procedure to fill the gap (HSC, 1989, para 4). However, these complaints may be being filtered through administrative procedures under the Hospital Complaints Procedure Act 1985. Given the pressures put on complainants and the imbalance of power between the patient and the NHS organization it is highly desirable that the HSC should have the power to examine complaints about clinical judgement without making himself judge on matters which only a professional can make. Research is beginning to emerge in this area which is likely to reinforce this argument.

The HSC has gone on record as saying that the hallmark of a service which cares for its consumers is an open complaints system which provides courteous, critical and thorough investigation of grievances. Each year the HSC investigates a substantial number of complaints about the way grievances were handled and upholds most of them. The record on the ground about the use of complaints or grievance procedures is very mixed. As already indicated although authorities are urged to monitor complaints and complaints procedures this is not done consistently. Complaints are not always examined for trends and systems weaknesses. This is not something which the HSC can do very effectively either without the power to investigate on his own initiative.

Additionally, the Hospital Complaints Procedure Act 1985 provides no direct enforcement mechanism for failure to implement its provisions. Presumably the requirements of the Act are enforceable through judicial review in the High Court. Whether these provide a reasonable remedy in all the circumstances is something that the HSC would have discretion about if a complaint referred to the absence of appropriate arrangements for implementation. Complaints which raise issues of general concern can be brought to the attention of the Parliamentary Select Committee by the Health Commissioner. The Committee can then require the health authority concerned to appear before them to give an explanation and answer questions. However, there is little evidence to suggest that the subsequent reports published by the Select Committee play a role in improving practice in health authorities other than those called before them.

In reality the HSC is able to examine a failure of administration. In spite of the improvements which he has managed to secure over the years the feeling is that something resembling a Code of Good Practice within the health service might be advantageous (Birkinshaw and Lewis, forthcoming). The twice yearly volumes of anonymized complaints which he submits to the appropriate ministers are extremely helpful. The HSC believes that these and the other reports produced prove useful not only as 'barometers of service quality' but as teaching material. As yet this is the only allusion to the issue of good practice that the HSC has made.

As regards his own operations the present Commissioner has pledged himself to do more about publicizing his office and has revised the general leaflet about his work to make it easier to follow and help people through the procedures involved in making a complaint to him. However, as Birkinshaw and Lewis (forthcoming) point out, although the matter of publicity is important, whilst ever the system is littered with exceptions to jurisdiction, increased publicity is only likely to lead to frustration and disappointment by those who had hoped they had found a champion but had found one 'fighting with one hand behind their back'.

CHALLENGE TO HEALTH CARE DECISIONS IN THE COURTS

The problems of the delivery of health services has come before the British courts in only a limited number of cases. Focal points for law and health have been most frequently concerned with liability for personal injury and medico-legal issues. Grievances about policy do not fit easily into the usual avenues for complaint. Consequently 'health law' has focused only rarely on the provision and allocation of services and the question of consumer rights under the public financing and regulation of the NHS.

Most of the cases cited below were precipitated by cuts made to health services as a result of constraints on financial resources. They are particularly notable for the lack of perceptive recognition in the judgements about the realities and complexities of health policy decision-making.

In R v Secretary of State for Social Services, the West Midlands Health Authority and the Birmingham Health Authority, *ex parte* Hincks 1980 the applicants, whose complaint was supported by members of the medical profession, had been on a waiting list for orthopaedic surgery for some years. Because of cuts in expenditure a scheme to improve orthopaedic services in the area, approved by the Department of Health in 1971, had had to be postponed indefinitely. A declaration was sought that the Secretary of State had failed to fulfil his duty under Section 3(1) of the National Health Service Act 1977 to provide a comprehensive health service. Counsel for the applicants argued that as there were no provisions in the present legislation limiting the expenditure of the Department of Health, it followed that if the Secretary of State needed money to carry out his duties then he must ensure that Parliament gave it to him. If Parliament did not, then a provision should be put into the statute excusing the minister from this duty.

In his judgement, Lord Denning M.R. pointed out that the minister's duty was not absolute; he had a discretion to evaluate financial resources as well to make decisions as to their allocation. Arguing that as funds were voted by Parliament the Health Service had to do the best it could with the total allocation. He added:

> The Secretary of State says he is doing the best he can with the
> financial resources available to him and I do not think he can be
> faulted on the matter.

Bridge L.J., whilst recognizing that the health service currently fell
far short of what 'everyone would regard as the optimum desirable
standard', declined to take the view that the courts had any role to
play in quality control. He hoped that the applicants had not been
encouraged to think that the court could enhance the standards of
the National Health Service, because 'any such encouragement
would be based upon manifest illusion.' The appeal was duly
dismissed.

In R v Central Birmingham Health Authority, *ex parte* Collier
1988 it was similarly argued that the RHA concerned, acting for the
Secretary of State, was in breach of a statutory duty to provide
treatment. Matthew Collier had been born in June 1983 with a heart
defect which had failed to be resolved by two previous operations.
At the time of the present case he was at the top of the waiting-list
for a further urgently required operation. However, as a result of a
shortage of intensive care beds, nurses and required after-care
treatment, the operation had been cancelled on three occasions.
The applicant sought leave for an order of certiorari and mandamus
in respect of the decision by the health authority not to conduct
heart surgery, despite numerous requests and an acceptance by the
health authority that there was an urgent need. The court's response was that it:

> could only intervene where it was satisfied that there was a
> prima facie case, not only of failing to allocate resources in the
> way which others would think that resources should be allo-
> cated, but of a failure to allocate resources to an extent which
> was 'Wednesbury unreasonable'.
>
> (Associated Provincial Pictures Houses v Wednesbury
> Corporation [1948] 1 KB 223)

In the instant case there was no such evidence. The Wednesbury
principle affirmed by the judiciary in this case is the classic formula
of the English courts that a policy can only be quashed if it is 'so
unreasonable that no reasonable body could have made it'.

Although Brown L.J. commented that there may be good
reasons or bad why the resources in this case did not allow all the

beds in the hospital to be used at the particular time, he did not enquire into those reasons.

Gibson L.J. stated that if he were in the same position as the applicant he would:

> want to be given answers about the supply to, and the use of, funds by this health authority. No doubt the health authority would welcome the opportunity to deal with such matters so that they could explain what the problems are.

But Gibson L.J. himself was not inclined to seek any comprehensive explanation in court. He added that the court:

> has no role of general investigator of social policy and of allocation of resources. Its jurisdiction . . . is limited to dealing with breach of duties under the law, including decisions made by authorities which are shown to be unreasonable.

Ex parte Collier followed R v Central Birmingham Health Authority, *ex parte* Walker 1987 in which the facts were almost identical. In that case Macpherson J. had held that the court had no jurisdiction to investigate:

> any case where the balance of available money and its distribution and use are concerned. Those are of course questions which are of enormous public interest and concern . . . but they are questions to be raised, answered and dealt with outside the court.

The above cases are important not only because they indicate the limited role which the courts see themselves as having in relation to the provision of health services to individuals but because they are instructive about the reality of challenging policy decisions in the British courts.

The response of the court in these cases was the assertion of the traditional role of ministerial responsibility and a restrictive interpretation of judicial review Wednesbury principles. There was a failure to acknowledge that decision-making about health care provision is in reality delegated far from the Secretary of State and Parliament, such that injustice may result from the opaque decision-making processes through which resource allocations are made.

It has already been argued that although consumer participation and accountability are implicit in the NHS decision-making structure, the channels for their practical implementation are as yet undefined and ineffective. The reliance of these judgments on accountability through Parliament, for the exercise of wide discretionary and delegated powers, serves only to ratify the opacity of decision-making rather than highlight the deficiencies which undermine the legitimacy of policy decisions. The result is that in cases of this nature the courts produce an extremely diluted and deferential standard of judicial review and weaken their own potential role in alleviating inconsistencies and structuring effective procedures for decision-making. As Harden and Lewis commented:

> Too often the judiciary appear to think that the ritual invocation of the Wednesbury test of reasonableness constitutes an adequate response to the need to define a role for the courts in maintaining rule of law values.
>
> (Harden and Lewis, 1986, p. 213)

If the courts in the instant cases had imposed on health authorities a duty to give a statement of the reasons and the evidence relied on for their decisions, the outcome for the individual applicants might well have been the same. But, at the least, the underlying assumptions of the true decision-makers might have been made more explicit and open to public assessment. The courts, quite rightly, are unwilling to determine the substance of health care policy, but that does not prevent them having a part to play in ensuring that decisions are taken in a reasoned and justified manner and that good standards for decisional processes are developed.

The foregoing argument, that the standard of judicial review associated with the Wednesbury test in the United Kingdom is inadequate to produce reasoned decision-making and that far more rigorous and demanding criteria are required, is supported by judicial experience in the USA.

LITIGATION AND HEALTH CARE REFORM IN THE USA

The history of attempts to instil democratic values into the American medical market is of particular interest for UK public lawyers concerned with examining different processes for the institutionalization of interest representation and accountability.

In the USA health care has always relied heavily on market forces, although this is increasingly modified by many regulations, programmes and tax incentives of both federal and state origin

(Enthoven, 1988). Services have been dominated by the medical profession and the hospital industry which largely determine the use, quality and price of services which may be funded from either public or private sources. This focus on medical provision through the market has had the effect to some extent of withholding from the pattern of health agency decision-making the development of 'due process' procedures which were evident in other areas of public policy (Rosenblatt, 1978).

However, the American courts on the whole perceive themselves as sharing responsibility with the legislature and executive for furthering general statutory and fundamental constitutional values. On occasion they have been much more clearly aware of the role they can play in the complex interaction between legislative provision, health agency response and judicial decisions than their British counterparts. In contrast to the results of litigation in the United Kingdom, several campaigns in the USA succeeded in re-orientating federal health care policy and increasing public involvement.

In the USA consumer groups have been able to use litigation as part of their strategy to increase overall awareness of health provision issues, altered health agency perceptions of their own role in allocating care, and increased the extent to which consumer interests were taken into account. The procedural techniques ultimately adopted required health authorities to make the facts and values in decision-making more explicit and stimulated improved forms of interest representation and accountability.

In order to realize the substantive aims of health care legislation, the American courts developed a consumer right, not to any specific level of services but to a process which defined and allocated resources in a way that could be justified and which provided a judicial remedy if this were not the case.

The legal techniques and strategy adopted were based on the 'hard look doctrine' devised in American administrative law. This doctrine aims to develop and maintain a standard of judicial review which seeks to ensure comprehensive analysis of policy options by decision-makers and the production of coherent reasons for action (Harden and Lewis, 1986, Chapter 9). This is notably in contrast to the soft standard of judicial review associated with the Wednesbury test, which has been adopted by the British courts and which, it has already been argued, has failed to promote an adequately reasoned pattern of decision-making in the policy process and supplement flagging democratic accountability procedures in the UK.

One of the campaigns conducted in the USA concerned the interpretation of the Hospital Survey and Construction Act 1946 (Blumstein, 1984). The Act was a small part of much wider proposals for the introduction of a comprehensive health care scheme which initially it was hoped would provide access to medical care for all USA citizens by linking public purposes to private means, a strategy which is increasingly used to implement social policy in the UK. The main aim of the Act was to identify long-term needs for hospital facilities and then provide finance for the necessary construction or modernization of hospitals.

Although basically a building programme, the Act importantly also contained very general provisions which laid down a requirement for equal access to health care. These were later to provide the vehicle for court action. Hospital facilities funded under the legislative provisions were to be available, without discrimination on account of race or religion to everyone residing in the area; and a reasonable volume of services were to be provided for those unable to pay, where the hospital's financial situation made this feasible.

Initial regulations made under the Act failed to specify any criteria for determining which patients were unable to pay or how a reasonable volume of free care should be measured. As a result, prior to 1972, the general provisions relating to equality of access were never enforced. But then a series of cases brought into effect the underlying rationale of the legislation, by successfully arguing that there should be better availability of hospital treatment to those not covered by any form of health insurance and that this necessitated detailed administrative policing.

A key case was Euresti v Stenner 1972 where it was held that the intention of the Act was to ensure that the poor would receive sufficient hospital services when needed. The court held that given the clear intent of the general provisions of the Act and the lack of administrative sanctions by the federal health authority, it was necessary and appropriate to infer a legal remedy to secure enforcement of the obligations of the hospitals involved.

Under pressure of continuous challenge in the courts from consumers, the federal health authority drafted regulations which defined a reasonable volume of care. However there was still a failure to monitor hospital compliance and in consequence many low-income patients continued to be refused treatment. Further litigation followed and in Newsom v Vanderbilt University 1978 the district court held that under the Act, uninsured, poor patients had a 'constitutionally protected right' to uncompensated hospital services and that any person denied care under its provisions was to be given:

> timely and adequate written notice of the reasons for denial, review by a decision-maker who had not participated in the initial finding on ineligibility, and a statement of reasons and the evidence relied on.

The courts were not claiming any authority to determine or expand the volume of resources available, but by regulating or overseeing the process by which statutory obligations were defined and administered the substance of health care policy in the USA was in part altered. Judicial recognition of the weakness of consumer power led to the imposition of procedural requirements and the eventual enactment of several important legislative provisions which aimed to ensure improved access to hospital services and which provided for both administrative and judicial enforcement.

The impact of economic constraints and the standard and availability of care in situations similar to those challenged in the British courts received judicial consideration in the USA in the two following cases (Annas *et al.*, 1990). In the first of these, Boone v Tate 1972, the findings of the court were similar to those in the Hincks and Collier cases.

The mayor of Philadelphia had authorized in December 1970 the dismissal of 550 employees from the Philadelphia General Hospital, the only municipal hospital in the city. Satisfactory hospital conditions, adequate facilities, proper care and staff were the direct responsibility of the hospital Board of Trustees, but the mayor had responsibility for shaping and controlling the city's fiscal policies and was under a general duty to prevent an occurrence of deficit in any fiscal year. Hence the curtailment of essential services. The order was challenged by patients who sought an injuction on the grounds that they were receiving inadequate care which they argued was a function not only of medical skills and technology but also of the financial duty of the city to provide those needs. There was no evidence that the city authority had failed to act in good faith, or had abused their discretion or acted for improper purposes.

The court held that although citizens had a right to expect adequate care, what constituted adequate medical care was an administrative decision taking into account not only medical opinion and standards but also financial resources available. In the light of prevalent financial conditions the plaintiffs had not established that they had been deprived of adequate care.

But then in the later case of Greater Washington DC Area Council of Senior Citizens v District of Columbia Government 1975, two local senior citizen organizations alleged inadequate treatment and facilities at the principal municipal hospital. The court found that facilities fell short of recognized and acceptable standards and were ordered to take appropriate action. The argument that had been put forward in Boone, that conditions were a product of fiscal constraints, was not accepted. The court instead demanded a clear demonstration that timely and positive efforts had been made to avert as far as possible a reduction in services and quality. They required a 'hard look' to be taken at policy decisions.

The issue is whether, given limits on resources, there is any alternative to accepting delivery of rationed care, or care that may well be substandard. Whilst in Boone the court held that given limits must be accepted, at least judicially, in Greater Washington the court held there was an alternative. Although the court had no power to order increased appropriations to the hospital, it ordered that existing resources should be used as effectively as possible and that this should be demonstrated openly. In affirming a higher standard of review the court recognized that injustice can arise through failures of management as well as underfunding. An acceptance of this line of argument by the British courts under the new arrangements for the separation of funding and provision could have interesting implications for the operation of NHS Trusts and the activities of health authorities.

Taken together the two campaigns mentioned resulted in a systematic scrutiny of health authority conduct. The emphasis of the American challenge to health agency decision-making was on the use of procedures as a means of giving substance to participatory requirements and the principles of openness and accountability. The American courts were prepared to raise the visibility of contested issues and increase the incentive for decisions to be more rational and accountable by determining the kind of procedure appropriate to achieve proper debate and scrutiny of policy in any given case. It is from this perspective that a strong case can perhaps be made for the subjection in the UK of wide discretionary powers to procedural requirements of the kind that have emerged in American administrative law.

In the UK the mechanisms to be developed would also depend on the context and significance of the issue or grievance. But at a minimum these would require health authorities and NHS Trusts to give notice of and acquire comment on suggested policy. Each body should then have to demonstrate openly that it had considered and weighed all relevant factors before finalizing a decision. Such an approach could begin to provide a surrogate means of involving the public in substantive health care choices. The imposition of procedural criteria could help reduce many of the perceived difficulties of institutionalizing interest representation and accountability, and it could also open up the possibility of a role for the courts in monitoring procedural quality through a stronger standard of judicial review than is presently the case.

CONCLUSION

The theme of this chapter has been that effective handling of grievances can be an important factor in accountability by monitoring the quality and provision of daily health care. Complaints may also contribute to management information and assist in the search for effectiveness and efficiency. Although health authorities are under a duty to establish complaints procedures these are, as yet, not fully developed. The potential of grievance redress in health management schemes is for the most part still under-recognized and receives a low priority. Although there are signs that this might be changing slowly, there is a long way to go before complaints are fully analysed and systematically fed into quality and policy processes.

Challenge to health care decisions in the courts has met with little success, although the litigation mentioned may have had a value beyond the individual results of the cases, by pushing policy issues to the forefront of public attention. However a much more effective solution would be for the courts to recognize the importance of evolving principles of good adminstration or management in health care, which sought to ensure a more comprehensive examination of policy options and a reasoned justification for action.

5

SOVEREIGN REMEDIES AND PREVENTIVE MEDICINE: PATIENT CHOICE AND MARKETS

MARKET TREATMENT

There is currently a deal of debate about the suitability of markets and competition and the role of regulation in public policy-making. The tension that exists between the desire to encourage the former and the need to protect wider public interests has very recently begun to manifest itself within health care provision. In contrast to other policy areas and perhaps contrary to popular belief 'marketization' of health care has failed to make much headway. This is most probably due to inherent restraints within the nature of health care itself. It is well known that as far as markets are concerned health care displays certain traits which militate against the market operating an equitable and efficient allocation of resources. In most countries, including the USA, the state has had to become involved in varying but mostly predominant degrees in the provision of health care in three main dimensions; in terms of access, in organizing finance, and in controlling delivery. Markets exist only at the margins for the delivery of certain services such as optics, pharmaceuticals or the contracting out of cleaning, catering and laundry (Moran, 1991).

In spite of this, the underlying assumption of recent developments in the NHS is that any 'imperfections' of market operations can be overcome. The optimum means of containing costs, increasing efficiency, improving quality and enhancing consumer sovereignty over health care decisions is seen to be by a momentum towards pro-market and pro-competitive strategies. The ideology is that competition, albeit structured, will stimulate the development of a system which would have the economic incentive and organizational capability to limit unnecessary services and develop new efficient patterns of care. It is also assumed that this framework will be sufficiently flexible to accentuate different values and combinations of services, in accordance with the needs and wishes of purchasers and consumers (Flynn, 1990).

Such an assumption needs to be carefully addressed. Whereas the right to health care is perceived as irreducible, the means of its provision are contingent. Only comprehensive empirical analysis of arrangements for the delivery of health care can indicate whether the right to it is being fully realized. The question must be asked under what conditions, if any, is the extension of an element of competition to more facets of health provision likely to improve the actual quality of care and whether or how far the operation and effects of what is generally termed a 'provider or internal market' are compatible with fundamental values, such as social choice and public accountability, inherent in democratic policy processes. Only then can the required regulatory framework be developed. For the public lawyer institutional design is a central concern and the issues that arise relate to legitimate processes for decision-making and the delivery of the expectations of the law-jobs.

Market proposals seek to promote the efficient use and delivery of resources and correct misallocation through competition and decisions based primarily on cost-benefit analysis. But the dynamics of competition in health care are at the very least unclear. Although competition may be instrumental in achieving efficiency under certain conditions, these are rarely articulated sufficiently to enable them to be incorporated into policy proposals. In addition, because of the lack of any clear philosophy and concept of health services, the meanings of cost and benefit are open to be interpreted to suit different and often very narrow purposes. The resultant information, although biased, is then presumed to reflect the accepted, general view.

In the market approach to health care cost is most frequently understood to mean a monetary equivalent. Benefit is also regarded as a quantifiable measure of treatment outcome such as the mortality rate, length of stay in hospital or chance of cure. In some contexts this will be adequate but it is rare for the conditions, contexts and purposes that justify these measures to be specified (Rosenblatt, 1981). This oversimplifies the way health care is experienced. 'Health' has a spectrum of meaning. Most basically it can be understood as the absence of disease and death and health care as a defence against both. Where this definition is accepted a particular clinical procedure can be evaluated in terms of monetary cost and in terms of the benefits of reduced disease and death rates. However, it should be noted that even these assessments are fraught with difficulties.

But health care can also be understood as a caring as well as a curative activity, its goals being to reduce pain and anxiety and increase the quality of life. The constitution of the World Health Organisation defines health as a 'state of complete physical, mental and social well-being and not merely the absence of disease or infirmity'. In some contexts there can be a conflict between the two aims. For example, high-technology equipment or drugs may delay death and reduce evidence of disease in a terminally ill patient in the first sense, but its iatrogenic effects may at the same time reduce the quality of life and undermine health care in its second sense (Enthoven, 1980; Rosenblatt, 1981).

Although advocates of the market approach recognize that modern health care has both a curing and a caring function, because the latter is very difficult to measure in any quantitative or statistical terms it is virtually excluded from cost-benefit analysis, even though such matters are likely to have a considerable effect on social organization and investment in health care provision. Until an holistic view can be taken of the effectiveness of clinical care and activity grounded more in a right to health care than being driven primarily by economic factors, it will be difficult for decision-makers to identify efficient use of resources, and misallocation will continue.

Much of the rhetoric about the new structure asserts that the market or an element of competition can play an important role in assuring health care quality. A primary means of ensuring quality is seen to be through the processes of contracting and bargaining for services between purchasers and providers. The notion is that the demands of purchasers will influence the provision of high-quality care. Hospitals or other providers that continually deliver unacceptable quality will face a declining demand for their services and will be thus induced to improve their quality to recapture business. However, as already discussed, improvements to quality depend very much on a nexus of interlinked factors, not least the ability to define and agree quality standards and the capacity to determine whether those standards are met.

Patients as ultimate consumers of health care are also to have a role in assuring quality by virtue of exercising greater choice in provision. However, the rhetoric of choice is much stronger than any explanation of how it is to be exercised (Klein, 1989). First of all there is little scope for the consumer to have any real choice at the point of entry into health care. The position of consumers of clinical care is not the same as that of consumers in other markets and the strategies that apply to the choice of other services or goods are only available to patients to a very limited extent. In fact there are few areas where the consumer is so ill-equipped to exercise their sovereignty. Some forms of care may be sufficiently recurrent to enable certain patients to make up their own minds as to whether they are receiving good quality care or they may be able to rely to some extent on the experience of friends or family. But since no two episodes that require medical care nor any two patients are alike these means carry inherent restrictions (Jost, 1988).

The scarcity of accurate information also plays a part in this situation. There is frequently no consensus of the value of some medical practices amongst doctors themselves making it more difficult for patients who lack technical knowledge to fully assess the quality of diagnosis and treatment and make rational choices. In addition, as most health services are required relatively quickly there is a limit on the extent to which the patient can 'shop around' to find the best services.

The ability of patients to make useful judgements about quality through their own experience and research is therefore extremely restricted. These very factors played a significant part in the rejection of a system of market allocation when the NHS was founded. In practice individual patient choices are surrogate ones made 'on trust' individually through the medical profession and collectively through purchasing DHAs.

But choice is also restricted at this level. In many areas the district hospital whether self-governing or managed, may have a near monopoly of service provision. It is unlikely that DHAs and GP fund holders will place many contracts further afield, other than those for highly specialized treatment. Although a proportion of care will inevitably be carried out in hospitals with which the DHA or GP does not have a contract, for example in the case of an emergency, there is to be no open-ended commitment on the part of district authorities to meet all non-contractual referrals. Even where there is no monopoly of provision there may be informal collusion between providers to limit certain services or providers may go for a 'least risk' selection of services rather than a more comprehensive one. Thus 'shopping around' and the exercise of choice may now be less of a possibility than under previous arrangements. This lack of consumer choice was recognized by Enthoven, the originator of the internal market concept who saw it as a major drawback (Enthoven, 1985).

As patients will always be dependent on those who provide care on their behalf, the fundamental issue is how this is to be regulated and how consumers can make their voice heard. The emphasis of current NHS reorganization is on individual choice and consumer sovereignty in the 'market'. But at a deeper level we are inevitably concerned with a wide range of more fundamental problems and responses to them from a social as well as individual perspective. These are issues of how best to get what is necessary to those who require it in an equitable as well as efficient manner. They are problems of collective choice and social enterprise, and the search for effective institutional design.

Doubts have already been expressed about the future role of CHCs in their present form as an adequate vehicle for public input into local health care provision. Consultation and public scrutiny are of particular importance in relation to the establishment and operation of NHS Trusts and in the new role of district authorities. But general concern about public accountability has been given little legislative recognition. This includes the disquiet from the Social Services Select Committee who recommended that urgent consideration be given to the ways in which the views of patients could be put before those involved in the planning and delivery of care.

The only concession to local involvement in the statutory framework for trusts is the requirement to appoint to Trust boards two 'community directors'. These are to be selected for the contribution they can make to the management of the hospital, not for any interest group they might represent. In addition Trusts are under no obligation to conduct any part of their business in open meetings. CHCs have no automatic right to attend routine meetings or receive documentary material relating to planning. Admission to such meetings is discretionary and may result in a cloak of 'commercial confidentiality' being put around Trust activities. It follows that a great deal of information about organization, forward planning and management objectives is unlikely to be open to public comment. In place of direct access to Trust business, CHCs are expected to deal with DHAs on matters relating to the provision and level of local services. But the structures for accountability are weak here too and CHCs are becoming increasingly dependent on the good-will of district health authority management (ACHCEW, 1991a). Without access to information as of right it will require outstanding perseverance on the part of CHCs to continue to represent the consumer diligently.

Currently, the exercise of collective choice comes far too late in the policy process and is based on too little information to be effective. Individual choice is then restricted at the point of entry to health care. Pollitt (1988) points out that consumerism in health provision is more about customer relations than any enhanced rights which entail true partnership or power sharing. The latter would require offering access to performance information of the sort that could be used to make the exercise of policy choices real and a framework to facilitate collective organization and represen-tation.

Planning guidance issued to RHAs for the year 1992–93 enables district purchasers to switch contracts for treatment to different hospitals where it is believed that this will provide better value for money and be in the interests of patients. To enable the Manage-ment Executive to intervene if it is considered that the future viability of a provider is likely to be in question RHAs are to inform the NHS ME of any proposed changes to contracting patterns in order to satisfy the Executive that the level of risk for providers and purchasers is manageable. This move may give a greater discretion to health authorities themselves to shop around on behalf of the public but it also signals a continuing commitment to market principles. As the trend towards a pro-competitive delivery of health care gathers momentum so the need for the following increases:

- More consideration of the conditions under which competition promotes choice and efficiency.
- Carefully designed mechanisms for service regulation and con-sumer sovereignty in the form of public accountability pro-cedures.

THE CITIZENS CHARTER

The major objective of recent policy to expand the capacity of patients to act as real consumers and require providers to function

on a commercial basis is reiterated by the inclusion of health services in the 'The Citizens Charter' (Cmd 1599) which aims to make
public services more answerable to their users and to raise overall
quality.

The general principles of the Charter are a declaration of what
every citizen is entitled to expect from public services. These include:

● Standards which are explicit, published and prominently displayed.
● There is to be a greater degree of openness, no secrecy about
  how public services are run, or how much they cost or who carries responsibility. Full and accurate information should be
  given about the services provided and targets to be met, together
  with audited information about results achieved. This should be
  in comparable form wherever possible.
● Those affected by services are to be consulted 'regularly and
  systematically' to inform decisions about what should be provided and management will be expected to demonstrate that
  user views have been taken into account in setting standards.
● There should be a well-publicized and readily available complaints procedure and code of practice for handling complaints.

Where possible there is to be an independent means of grievance
review. Where internal complaints procedures fail and the body
complained against has not settled a grievance in a satisfactory
manner, the government is considering the introduction of a
scheme of lay adjudicators to deal with minor claims. Rather than
make provision for compensation where there are serious problems the government intends to introduce new forms of redress
which will aim to stimulate efficiency rather than divert funds from
service improvement. New avenues of redress under consideration
for the NHS are a provision for treatment to be carried out by
other providers where, for example, guaranteed waiting times fail
to be met, and an arbitration system as a simpler and quicker
avenue for resolution of claims of medical negligence. Commitment to raising standards and implementation of these principles is
to be firmly planted at the local level in line with government
policy to devolve decision-making and responsibility from central
management.

Building on current NHS reforms Patients Charters are being
produced which aim to set out what the NHS should provide and
what patients are entitled to expect from health services. A

national Patients Charter already specifies ten individual guaranteed rights:

- To receive health care on the basis of clinical need, regardless of ability to pay.
- To be registered with a GP.
- To receive emergency medical care at any time.
- To be referred to a consultant where necessary.
- To be given a clear explanation of any treatment proposed, including any risks and available options.
- To have access to health records (although this only applies to records made after 1 November 1991).
- To withhold consent to treatment or participation in medical research or student training.
- To be given detailed information about local health services, including quality standards and maximum waiting times.
- To be guaranteed admission for treatment by a specific date no later than two years from the day when the patient is placed on a waiting-list.
- To have any complaint about health services investigated and to receive a prompt reply from the chief executive or general manager.

The Patients Charter also introduces nine public service principles which are not legal rights but specific standards which the NHS is expected to achieve as 'circumstances and resources' allow. These are:

- Respect for privacy, dignity, religious and cultural beliefs.
- Provision for those with special needs, such as physical and mental handicap, to be able to use health services without difficulty.
- Provision of information to relatives and friends, subject to the wishes of the patient.
- Standard times, waiting times for ambulance services, initial assessment of what is required in accident and emergency departments and out-patient appointments.
- Less frequent cancellation of operations.
- A named qualified nurse, midwife or health visitor responsible for each patient.
- Improved coordination of discharge arrangements.

From April 1992 health authorities will be expected to produce local charters specific to their own services which set out and publicize the main standards of service negotiated with hospitals and other providers. These are to be widely available and prominently displayed. Although the government does not regard it to be sensible to set national quality standards because of variations in local circumstances, guidance is to be given by the NHS Management Executive on the main areas in which local standards of service must be established, monitored and published to provide a consistent national basis. Guidance has already been issued on maximum waiting times for treatment and specific, timed appointments for all out-patient visits. A list of performance indicators to be published will be included in the national patient charter. Clear information about primary health care services is also to be available, each general practice being required to detail the services offered.

The government also states an intention to strengthen the impact of audit and regulation to open up the way for quality improvements. Proposed legislation will require the Audit Commission to publish league tables of health authority performance, although there is as yet no mention of health authorities being required to publish a response to auditor reports, as will be the case with local authorities.

The scope of competitive tendering in the NHS is also to be extended to cover such services as distribution, warehousing, non-emergency transport, document transfer and management services. The government believes that tendering has already raised standards of performance and made substantial savings, but procedures have in the past been extremely complex and placed obstacles in the way of private sector tenders (but see Wood, 1988). The contracting process is consequently to be simplified and streamlined. Tender documents in the future are only to describe and set out the standard of service required. They will not be expected to specify how that standard is to be achieved, as this is seen by government to stifle innovation and enterprise and deter potential tenderers.

The principles and initiative of the Citizens and Patients Charter are to be welcomed; as the government itself has stated, 'quality does not happen by accident, improvement requires reform, innovation and tough decisions'. The question is whether the Charter will in practice deliver a better deal for the public and fulfil the opportunity to empower them as citizens, or whether it will merely reinforce the public as customer with very limited capacity to influence policy decisions. Much depends on the quality of the mechanisms and procedures developed to give substance to the Charter principles and the significance attached to those procedures by those responsible for their implementation and monitoring. These factors will influence whether or not the Charter and indeed other reforms turn out to be 'light or heavyweight' in their effect.

Although a step in the right direction the overall tenor of the Charter is primarily one of individual rights in the doctor–patient relationship and a continuing emphasis on the individualization of choice which, it has been argued, are limited. Many of the provisions in the Patients Charter are not new, they have been operative for some time, but have not been given the requisite publicity. The suspicion must be that given other recent changes to NHS democratic processes, even the principle of consultation is likely to amount to no more than a requirement to conduct 'customer surveys' about hospital support services and are unlikely to involve any consideration of policy matters. Most patients are likely to continue to be remote or even entirely absent from crucial decisions on the actual supply and delivery of services (Flynn, 1990). Those decisions are made by largely unrepresentative, and for the most part publicly unaccountable health authorities, acting as advocates, through internal and *ex parte* organizational bargaining processes.

As ACHCEW point out, for patients to be empowered by exercising real choice and participating fully in health care it is essential that they have access to information about the quality of local services and available options (1991b, p. 1). But doubts must be expressed about the quality of information to be published in health authority league tables. These seem likely to indicate comparison of supply costs or waiting times of which limited use can be made by consumers where their capacity for choice is inherently restricted. Furthermore, cost effectiveness and faster throughput rates are no indication of better quality.

The rights and standards of the Patients Charter are designed to meet the commitments of the Citizens Charter, and the NHS will play a full part in the Chartermark scheme when it is launched. CHCs will inevitably be involved in local monitoring of standards, in publicizing Charter standards and in assisting patients to enforce their rights. ACHCEW argues that it would therefore be logical for CHCs to be consulted on the awarding of Chartermarks and to be able to nominate health services for the award. Recent NHS reforms have already been made increasing demands on CHC resources but no increases in funding have been forthcoming. If the commitment to 'independent validation of performance against standards' is a serious one additional resources need to be made available to CHCs (ACHCEW, 1991, p. 20).

The danger is that consideration of outcomes will be nothing more than superficial and information systems will remain based on simple criteria, focused mainly on quantifiable results, unconcerned with institutional processes and the dynamics of provider–purchaser relations except as they are influenced by economic incentives.

For anyone committed to equality of access, public participation, accountability and improved quality in health care the initial impression gained from much of the rhetoric of the recent reforms, Citizens Charter and market literature is one of shared values and of familiar and worthy goals. On closer examination this soon disappears. This is because these values and goals are likely to be achieved with a minimum of public involvement in decision-making and inadequate procedures for public accountability.

In short, politics in its truest and broadest sense is missing from the structure of the NHS. And yet because of the basis of funding of the NHS, notwithstanding the significance of health to society, its administration and management will always be inextricably political. The balance of power may be currently adapting or shifting internally, but it is health authority and hospital management (and this may include clinicians) who have had their scope of control extended by the processes of contracting and of management-defined efficiency and effectiveness. None of this has improved the position of patients as citizen. When the long traditions of professional dominance and public ineffectiveness are properly considered the chances of success of a market approach adjusting the balance between providers or purchasers and the consumer appear unlikely, particularly in the face of evidence that markets in health care merely reproduce difficulties similar to those already experienced under other administrative arrangements (Maynard, 1987). This makes the need for alternative conceptions of public management and the means of their facilitation critical. The aim should be to move away from managerial orthodoxy to develop a brand of management that recognizes that public service goes much deeper than meeting the needs and wishes of the consumer at a superficial or rhetorical level; it is more about making services accessible, equitable and publicly accountable (Metcalfe and Richards, 1987).

Although much of the debate about the organization of the NHS has centred on the introduction of market and competition elements through active state intervention, these should be seen in the wider context of a whole set of developments to which some significance should be attached. The changes to health services mirror developments that have been taking place throughout central government. In 1988 the government launched a major initiative in civil services management in response to an Efficiency Unit report, *Improving Management in Government: the Next Steps*. As part of a drive towards more businesslike and decentralized delivery of public services, the executive functions of central government are being handed over to Next Steps agencies, of which there are already more than 50. The intention is that where practicable all executive activities will be operating along these lines by the end of 1993.

As with the changes to the NHS one of the aims of the reforms is to give a new sense of direction and a sense of pride in the services provided. The challenge is to establish responsive, consumer-orientated services which meet the reasonable expectations of the public whilst being efficient and cost effective. Although not Next Steps agencies, the structure and principles underlying the operation of the NHS Management Executive and health authorities are very similar. There are no blueprints for Agencies as it is intended their structure and operation should reflect their own specific requirements. But several key concepts and mechanisms are reflected in the organization of the NHS and most agency operations.

These can be summarized as firstly, a clarification within government departments of activities concerned with policy development and those concerned with executive activity and their organization as substantially autonomous units, whilst remaining within the parent department. Secondly, a shift of emphasis from control of processes to more control through accountability for results. Thirdly, a clearer specification of the results to be achieved through the setting of specific service and financial targets and finally the appointment of a Chief Executive who has scope to deploy resources flexibly to meet objectives and is personally accountable for results. To meet these aims each agency has a published framework document which states the job to be done, the lines of responsibility and the extent of managerial independence. Through this and the corporate and annual plans that support it, targets for standards of service and budgets are set.

None of these developments are wholly novel in many areas of public policy. The NHS, for example, has been moving towards a system of performance review designed to monitor progress towards the achievement of very specific targets since the early 1980s. As Klein has pointed out, these moves reflected the general emphasis of government policy expressed in the Financial Management Initiative and the commitment to reducing public spending and a growing preoccupation with value for money (Klein, 1989, p. 205).

Given that the new structures have been developed against the traditional background of inadequate measures for public accountability which it is argued here are a precondition of the achievement of public goals and purposes, and the often disappointing results and difficulties which beset earlier initiatives the question arises whether it is possible to identify any ways in which the new structures might promote an 'in-built dynamic for better performance' which go beyond those former attempts in the NHS (Hickey, 1989).

The immediate effect of re-establishing two central boards of the NHS in the guise of the Policy Board and Management Executive was the necessity to clarify respective roles and responsibilities. Whether this works in operation remains to be seen, but the dynamics of accountability are still unclear and appear to be far from simple. The continuing and direct contact between politicians and health authorities is at odds with the rhetoric of local responsibility for decision-making and is a manifestation of the persistence of public accountability through the Secretary of State to Parliament. On the other hand if too great a gap opens between those formulating policy and those executing it at a local level this could also be damaging. It is therefore crucial that communication and consultation should continue so that realistic benchmarks for operation can be set (Harden and Lewis, 1986). The separation of funding from provision should help clarify the new role for DHAs, that of taking responsibility for specifying standards and monitoring their achievement. Previously this responsibility had fallen to those who were actually delivering the service. Accountability is more likely to have some genuine meaning where it falls outside those actually providing the service (but see the section on the role of contract and see Harden, 1992).

The potential advantages of setting objectives and performance targets are great, the underlying philosophy and success of the RMI rests on the provision of clear objectives. Yet within the health service there is a long way to go in delivering service targets and linking them explicitly to resource objectives, not only because of the lack of data, information systems and technology but because such changes of culture need careful nurturing to eliminate sectional interests.

On the positive side, contracting has had the effect of encouraging health authorities to clarify priorities and may have instilled a sense of purpose which in time may produce more dynamic and innovative management. Another result of the emphasis on performance priority and target setting might be to raise the expectations of the public and make explicit and subject to argument what was once implicit, and therefore largely uncontroversial. The gains for the public may therefore be greater than at first expected.

The importance also of the psychological factor in motivating action for improved services should not be underestimated. But it is important that its implications should not be applied solely for the benefit of management; incentives need to be identified for all interested parties. For the goal of public accountability this amounts to real opportunities to influence policy processes. At present DHAs may appear to engage in consultation but, as has already been argued, this is often cursory because of inadequate procedures and a lack of means to guarantee quality of consultation, so that in effect the main lines of policy development lie elsewhere.

Stewart (1981) argues that all interested parties need to believe that their interests lie in co-operation and identifies three requirements to strengthen incentive for all parties to participate in good faith:

1 Delay to decisions induced by successive rounds of comment should be reduced as far as possible. This includes avoiding excessive regulation and judicial oversight. The central task for law is to encourage and facilitate rather than intimidate and regulate (Harden and Lewis, 1986, p. 289).
2 Health authorities must be prepared to give up a measure of control over policy processes and allow access to active participation at an earlier and more flexible stage of policy making.
3 To participate more effectively in these less formal processes interested parties, particularly those that act on behalf of the consumer such as CHCs, need better access to information and to adequate funding.

CONCLUSION

The changes to the organization of the NHS discussed in this chapter have been designed to introduce an element of competition into health care, the intention being to improve the quality and efficiency of provision. But, it has been argued that despite rhetoric to the contrary the potential influence of the public in these new developments is marginal, not only because of the scarcity of information but also because of the imprecise nature of medicine itself. Choice is in reality restricted at an individual and at the collective level. Although the Patients' Charters are to be welcomed they can only be regarded as a beginning and are unlikely in their present form to bring about any significant change. The fundamental need is to develop the Charters into specific rights which can bring about a reorientation of the current culture of lack of accountability.

If, as was argued in the first chapter, we aspire to build our public organizations on democratic principles there needs to be a recognition that the stakes all participants have in health care require appropriate *ex ante* and *ex post* accountability processes. Recent developments are seeking to spread the responsibility for health costs and quality such that the whole issue of health care begs a constitutional framework which encourages the development of performance evaluation of all constituents and better communication of the considerations taken into account in formulating health policy. This is fundamental to improvement in the quality of health care for it is not possible to look critically at how to achieve optimum provision without considering how the organization of health care itself can have a real effect on choice and accountability.

Market mechanisms, particularly those characterized by poor information, and an emphasis on economic accountability are unlikely to solve the major problem of the NHS which is that of producing an equitable, high-quality and efficient service. Structured competition is in reality merely an adminstrative means of stretching limited resources, it should not be regarded as a substitute for reasoned health care policy and planning. However, a by-product of pro-competitive structure and contracting for services may be an impetus towards a realization of genuine quality assessment systems. Whether such an incentive could have arisen without the implementation of the contract mechanism is a different question. However, some promising avenues have been opened up which could point the way to improving health care as long as these are properly monitored and overall objectives as opposed to purely financial ones are made explicit.

6

PROGNOSIS AND PREVENTIVE MEDICINE: ANTIDOTES, TONICS AND LEARNING

The organization of our health care provision is once again in a state of upheaval. At its inception the structure of the NHS incorporated a miscellaneous alliance of private, municipal and charitable health provision. Yet since that time, the recurring difficulties of reconciling public accountability with other often diverse interests which manifest themselves in the structure of the NHS and have contributed to three major reorganizations in recent years, have received sparse academic consideration.

In particular the British legal system and public law has made little contribution to the development of any formula of what can be termed administrative or organizational 'due process'. Fuelled and misled by the myth of public accountability through the answerability of government to Parliament, public law has 'fallen victim to changed circumstances' and has failed to come to terms with the requirements of surrogate political processes and to facilitate a rational foundation for decision-making. Consequently public law has failed to give due consideration to that problem of the management of public institutions.

The analysis in this book rests on a firm belief in the importance of a proper constitutional underpinning for all public activity. Because, by its very nature public power is exercised on behalf of all citizens, everyone has a right to participate in and express concern with its application. The challenge for society and the designers of its public institutions is to provide a means to draw together and manage those diverse and sectional interests so as to safeguard the citizen as an individual and a member of society from arbitrary decisions. It is now essential to look beyond the traditional forms of accountability to a transformation and regeneration of a productive role for administrative law (Harden and Lewis, 1986, pp. 224, 240).

The NHS like other public organizations has tended to look increasingly to technical and professional solutions to its difficulties. At the same time its mechanisms for public accountability have failed to adapt to these changes, leaving the way open for incremental and reactive conduct based on an inadequate analysis and superficial debate of options. And yet public accountability is at the heart of the relationship between consumers and the providers of health services and the organization of the NHS is still based on an assumption of accountability for all its constituent groups, from politicians, to management to medical professionals.

Such a focus should serve to enhance to a significant degree the process of social choice in health care delivery. But in the NHS, like other areas of social welfare objectives are currently sought to be achieved through means and forms of management more characteristic of private corporate enterprise. These characteristics of modern governmental institutions have gone hand in hand in the NHS with and a down-grading of participative citizenship and an espousal of consumerism, through an attempt to develop a market within government administration. But the concepts of social choice and social justice have implications which go beyond individual selection and consumption and self-determination (Rosenblatt, 1981). The forms of management and the brand of consumerism currently being infused into our public institutions have nowhere yet been demonstrated to be superior, so that it is essential that their shortcomings as well as their virtues need to be constantly examined.

It is not argued here that there should be a reversal of current developments in health care. Rather, the aim is to ensure that structured competition and the provider market is publicly accountable and properly policed to ensure quality information is not withheld and that the social values which are sought to be protected are neither solely nor even primarily concerned with cost containment. Public accountability necessitates procedures for the open discussion of priorities and objectives before decisions reach a stage where there is no real choice. It also demands justification of policy choices and channels for the expression of dissatisfaction and the redress of grievances. Accountability is an ongoing evaluative process which should provide a vehicle for improvement and change. Such a focus might preclude the provision of any easy answers, but it should frame the questions that could lead to a better

understanding of contending issues. Accountability is thus fundamental to an organization's learning. For this to become a possibility some external direction is required and the recurrent theme
throughout this book is that the techniques and processes of law can
assist in providing that external direction.

Legal procedures, posited by the law-jobs, can offer a model of
public management where authority can be supported by construc-
tive criticism and improved by its ability to respond to the needs of a
better informed public. This is the constitutional basis of public
service which needs to be the focus of government. The responsibility for its facilitation lies with the political and legal system.

In the NHS the law-jobs are present to a greater or lesser extent
through the many facets of its organizational structure. But it
should be clear from discussion in the previous chapters that the full
potential of the law-jobs has not yet been realized and there is some
deficit in the operation of all four.

CHOOSING GOALS AND OBJECTIVES

The choice of priorities and objectives are essentially political
decisions and occur within the NHS from governmental level
through the health authorities to the local level. The actual processes of policy decisions are still by no means clear. The organization of the NHS has sought to maintain a traditional distinction
between policy formation and implementation with scant recognition in the development of its structure that the impact of policy is
frequently affected as it is mediated through the institution and
those working within it. Policy can be selectively interpreted and
distorted at all levels as attempts are made to reconcile and overcome perceived pressures and difficulties. Such action is not made
explicit through the current structures for policy making in the
NHS, and there is little opportunity for competing objectives to be
discussed. This is because there is a lack of relevant information and
forums for managing debate about potential options. The current
focus on financial viability and strategy and the consequent information provided to meet this emphasis leave little room for attention to be given to wider social and even clinical values. The impact
of the NHS Policy Board at governmental level and the role of
DHAs in deciding priorities and objectives in their localities need to
be carefully researched and addressed before the problems attend-
ant in trying to reconcile a centrally funded and policy orientated

organization with delivery which corresponds to needs at a local level can be solved. It is crucial that policy decisions be opened up to assist analysis so that lessons can be learned and efforts made to develop mechanisms to put things right.

THE ALLOCATION OF DECISION-MAKING AUTHORITY

At government level a mix of personnel and cultures from government, the health service, commerce and industry form the membership of the NHS Policy Board. Although this could, if not discouraged, produce a range of interesting views and bargaining complexities, all non-executive members were appointed for their known support of the present focus in the provision of health care. Below that level decision-making authority encompasses primarily management staff and medical professionals. Although the aim is stated to be to devolve as much decision-making as possible to a local level, the emergence of this in practice is questionable. The need by the NHSME to oversee overall expenditure is likely to continue to constrain health authority autonomy. Chapter 2 also indicated that there has been a progressive exclusion of the public or the representatives of the public from decision-making as the emphasis on decisions being taken by those with more business-oriented skills has increased.

PREVENTIVE CHANNELLING

The latest changes have confirmed encouraging moves towards policy and priority review in both the management and clinical setting, by the introduction of measures including resource management and medical audit. These could provide an excellent opportunity to widen the scope of public input and accountability if their focus as a management activity were reorientated. We need to ensure that information gleaned from monitoring is put to use for wider purposes than purely economic considerations. New health developments are likely to increase the number of *ex parte* communications, due to the demand for greater information and knowledge.

It is therefore likely that the variety of pressure groups and professional organizations that exist in relation to health care will be increasingly drawn into the shadowy field of policy analysis (Harden and Lewis, 1986, pp. 241–2; McLachlan, 1990). It is important that this occurs in a structured and visible way, so that inevitably biased information can be exposed and properly assessed and formal procedures are not outflanked by covert, informal negotiation. The development of accountability measures can help ensure that a hard look is taken at policy options and proposals, something which is not guaranteed under present arrangements.

RESOLUTION OF DISPUTES

Channels for the expression and proper resolution of grievances are a prime aspect of accountability and can be an indirect factor in consumer input to policy decisions. The moves towards the better internal handling of health service complaints are to be welcomed, but there is still room for improvement. A positive culture of a right to express dissatisfaction has not yet been established. Whether more substance will be given to this as a result of the Patients and Citizens Charters remains to be seen. But the latter might have the effect of raising the visibility and increasing public awareness of what is or is not being provided in our health service and give rise to legitimate expectations that consumer views on these matters should be taken into account. Where provision falls below published standards the courts may possibly take a different view from that stated in cases cited in Chapter 4.

Organizations, like people, need to learn to be able to develop and mature. Properly designed, the law-jobs can assist all groups concerned with the provision of health care to establish their identity, resolve conflict, and set norms of practice such as openness and co-operation.

Procedures need to be developed which sustain a rigorous analysis of all policy options including those affecting unrepresented or inarticulate groups so that vital issues are neither unmentioned nor go without their due consideration. The debate engendered would be a critical and extensive source of knowledge and provide the opportunity for improvement that learning encompasses to put things right. The regulatory framework envisaged needs to be clear enough to give guidance and resilient enough to withstand subsequent developments but must not inhibit flexibility. This is a form of law known as 'soft or reflexive law' which structures or restructures semi-autonomous organizations by designing their procedures for both internal and external conduct and coordination (Teubner, 1983, p. 255; Harden and Lewis, 1986, pp. 293–7). Through these means communication and learning between interested parties are facilitated at all stages of the policy process. Only when these processes have been successfully put in place will the organization of the NHS be able to reach maturity and be moved towards an optimum performance level. Where these concerns are insufficiently addressed the organization's learning and maturing process can be driven below ground resulting in covert politicking, hidden agendas and abuse of power. In short concealed conduct disrupts standard setting and subverts performance.

PUBLIC MANAGEMENT AND THE LAW-JOBS

The underlying premiss of the current reorganization was stated to be a decentralization of decision-making power and a concomitant increase in local level autonomy for the provision and operation of health services (*Working for Patients*, 1989). However, on closer inspection the reforms are arguably primarily concerned with extending the predominance of the particular forms of management processes in health care provision already mentioned. There is as yet, notwithstanding the provisions of the Patients Charter, little new institutional machinery to suggest that improved standards accountability that go beyond a concern for economic efficiency will be fostered, and so enable the continual evaluation of services which are responsive to public as well as provider and management assessment of needs.

Without doubt modern policy processes require increased and improved management skills in both policy development and execution, but these need to be developed within their specific contexts. Institutional arrangements also need to ensure that these do not become annexed to a system which encourages ill-planned, reactive and unaccountable action, rather than conduct that is continually shaped by the context and specific purposes of the organization (Ranson and Stewart, 1989). For the latter to have a possibility of becoming a reality – in this case the facilitation and maintenance of an accountable and legitimate system of health care which is genuinely responsive to public needs and values – an accommodation between the techniques of public law and those of a modified view of the undertakings of public management is essential.

The main concern is that the distinctive features of public affairs are managed in such a way that they are acclaimed rather than marginalized. The introduction of any revised concept of public management is of course problematic. Sound public management, the potential to recognize and then deal with the changing complexities of public organizations, necessitates the development of new skills and awareness. This is not something that can be 'conjured from thin air'. It requires a change in culture and a revision of established preconceptions about management and its relationship with accountability. Such changes require solid foundations and sufficient resources with which to build, as both management and accountability systems can be no better than their building fabric allows.

One solution should by now be obvious, that is to ground our conception of public management in the law-jobs which 'contribute to our democratic ideals and to the optimization of resource allocation' by offering a range of means with which to shape and mould collective matters (Lewis, 1981). From the perspective that our democratic expectations require that public organizations should be wholly accountable, the correlation between a proper role for public management (one that enhances public interests and access to decision-making) and the law-jobs is clear. The sum total of the law-jobs amounts to the theory and discipline of public management.

Recent debate about the nature of public management has aimed to clarify and expand its definition and to find a concept which successfully encompasses the distinctive elements of a public organization (Stewart and Clarke, 1987). Management has been defined generally as taking responsibility for the performance of a system. This is stated to include 'all phases of the policy process and their coordination to achieve overall policy purposes' (Metcalf and Richards, 1987, pp. 35–42).

The role of public managers is to develop a capacity to cope effectively with ambiguities, conflicts and potential instability of organizations and to recognize that accountability procedures are operated, implemented and sometimes manipulated by those within the system. This requires training and a re-orientation of the perceptions of present management objectives. Effective public management can then be defined in terms of innovativeness, adaptability, and a capacity to learn and manage change (Ranson and Stewart, 1989, pp. 19–24). Stress is therefore laid on management as a responsive, flexible and adaptive process which can

Law-jobs	Legitimacy and accountability	Public management skills
		Enabling functions
1 Allocation of decision-making authority. Development of structural and administrative framework. Discretion and delegation of business.	← Right to manage →	(a) Innovation. (b) Information gathering, problem formulation, generation of solution. (c) Developing policies to achieve existing objectives and prompt strategic changes.
2 Choosing goals and objectives.	← Flexibility and adaptability →	(d) Integration, coordination complementary to innovation.
3 Implementation of policy and monitoring: preventive channelling	← Feedback →	(e) Cooperation and support.
4 Disposition of the trouble case.	← Stability →	*Maintenance functions* Interpreting and applying general principles to particular situations and working within policy parameters.
		Post decision phase and implementation.
		Resolution of disputes monitoring.

Figure 6.1   Conduct of public business

develop a range of options for both system-enabling and system maintenance functions.

However, in an organization where management involves matters which stem from public purposes, values and conditions, these skills must be set against a constitutional and political backcloth. The task is to 'support citizenship and government' (Ranson and Stewart, 1989, p. 19). In this respect the law-jobs provide the means of underpinning public management with the democratic principle of accountable decision-making by the provision of a blueprint for legitimate institutional design (Figure 6.1). Public management activities, like public law techniques, are thus recognized as complementary surrogate political conduct with a potential to reinforce a commitment to accountability as an operational norm, through the designing of appropriate patterns of action between the organization and those who require access to policy processes.

INDEPENDENT REVIEW

The very nature of accountability dictates that the initiative must be held by those who question the decisions being taken. That initiative relies ultimately on the independent generation of information. Whilst health authorities are bodies with a potential for generating debate and testing critical assumptions and providing an opportunity to make creative use of planning evaluation, because of their many competing interests and allegiances they cannot be relied upon to respond effectively to consumer or more correctly citizen concerns. As the NHS becomes more fragmented and pluralistic, and the division between public and private provision becomes blurred, the latter requires an intermediary body to perform a less diverse role between providers and users. CHCs with an expanded remit would be admirably placed to fufil the task.

At the Parliamentary level also careful consideration should be given to the range of constituencies required to act as public watchdog both for and through Parliament. Harden and Lewis (1986) point to the gaps in current accountability mechanisms and evaluative arrangements which beg the need for some independent assessment machinery that will have relevance for decisions on national policies. They and other commentators suggest intermediary advisory bodies which could be specifically placed both to report to Parliament and be consulted by it and which can take an overall view of what is required (see also McLachlan, 1990).

What is really being advocated is the development of quality control measures for decision-making. Because of the limitations of budget, personnel and time and of course relationship with the Secretary of State for Health the NHS Policy Board and the Management Executive cannot hope to develop in-house all the information and specialized experience needed to make effective insights and non-biased judgements. The use of an advisory body – outside the executive and capable of spanning the area of potential conflicts between medical, management and social requirements – is a possible solution to the problem of presenting more diverse views and perspectives to the public and to Parliament. In the USA extensive use has been made of advisory committees which have provided federal agencies such as the Food and Drug Administration (FDA) with the resources to carry out reviews that could not otherwise have been accomplished (Stewart, 1981, pp. 1355–6).

In the UK it has been suggested that some version based on the model of the Social Security Advisory Committee (SSAC) could provide scope for extending public accountability and instituting a policy dialogue with decision-makers being required to justify any departures from advisory body recommendations (Harden and Lewis, 1986, pp. 253–5). The Secretary of State is obliged to consult the SSAC on proposals for a wide range of regulations and to consider any report and recommendations made by the Committee. The Minister is also required to lay a copy of SSAC reports before Parliament and explain how far effect has been given to them and give reasons for not following recommendations. A similar body could have potential to provide Parliament with a 'hard look' standard of information through its centrality to policy making and it constitutional arrangements.

However, the usefulness of advisory committees may be limited where extensive amounts of data must be gathered and basic research undertaken as in the case of the health policy and standard setting. Although there are a considerable number of institutions which carry out research in the health care field it has often been difficult to co-ordinate and link their work. As McLachlan (1990) has stated:

> what we should be seeking are the continuing means for objective judgment on health care arrangements and policies.
>
> (McLachlan, 1990, p. 207)

Klein points to the uncertainty of health policy and the importance of devising organizational structures that can readily adapt to rapidly changing circumstances. In doing so he too underscores the organization of health care provision as a learning process. Policy judgements and parliamentary assessments therefore need to be based on comprehensive and informed evaluation. To this end the establishment of an Institute of Health has been canvassed and is worthy of serious consideration. In the past it has been suggested that the brief of the Health Advisory Service could be broadened to cover overall aspects of health care for public discussion.

The Health Advisory Service (HAS) was set up in 1969 to act as an inspectorate for hospitals and services for the mentally handicapped, mentally ill, elderly patients and the chronically sick. Acute and family practitioner services are excluded from its remit. The HAS is operationally independent from the Department of Health and the NHS and provides 'a reporting service for the Secretary of State' (Klein and Hall, 1974). Klein and Hall support the view that an inspectorate with an advisory and regulatory role would be a direct source of information to the Department of Health and provide a framework for national information into which to fit local concerns, demands or complaints.

It is unlikely that the newly established Clinical Standards Advisory Group (CSAG) which was established at the insistence of the House of Lords, to allay the fears of the royal colleges that clinical standards might suffer through the operation of the 'internal market', will fulfil the purpose, at least as presently constituted (Sheldon, 1991). The key function of the CSAG will be to guarantee and improve clinical standards by the provision of independent advice to the Secretary of State and the NHS Management Executive. The House of Lords envisaged the body as having a wide remit to advise, carry out studies and submit reports on issues relating to standards of care at national, regional and local levels at the request of the Minister.

The Group's programme is to be decided between it and the Secretary of State, taking into account suggestions by health authorities and other organizations such as the royal colleges. However, doubts exist about the independence of the CSAG and the extent and interpretation of its powers. It is not clear whether the Group will be able to investigate aspects of clinical quality on its own initiative or whether its reports will be publicly available. It has been stated that it will have neither an inspectorate nor accreditation function, with the result that its remit is not even as wide as that of the HAS. Although members, appointed on the recommendation of the royal colleges, see the CSAG as having a role similar to that of the Audit Commission in relation to clinical standards, much will depend on the lead given by the chair. In order to act truly independently and set a new standard of public accountability the CSAG would need to include non-professional representatives, have additional powers to consider ethical and social implications of health policy and be given more extensive resources.

McLachlan (1990) has suggested that the Institute of Medicine of the National Academy of Sciences in Washington D.C. (IOM) could provide a model whose form and objectives could be adapted to British purposes. The Institute was set up to try to clarify and offset problems which were being experienced in the USA in the provision of health care because of increasingly heavy demands on health services and their complex relations with other sectors of public policy. Recognizing that the problems of health care and service delivery are so large that their solution requires the competence and concern of disciplines other than medicine the Institute is broadly based. Its 500 active members are elected from health, medical and biological sciences and other related fields such as behavioural and social sciences, administration, law and engineering. In operation it is an apolitical body capable of objective analysis of issues for recommending policy in all aspects of health care and its delivery. Members and non-member experts serve on committees for the study of critical health issues, without compensation. The issues which the Institute addresses may be identified by Congress, the executive, various foundations and other private sector organizations or by the IOM itself. The IOM is governed by an elected council of 21 members and is organized into operating divisions dealing with health sciences policy, health promotion and disease prevention, health care services, mental health and behavioural medicine and international health. The IOM oversees a programme of some 60–70 research projects at any given time.

Within the UK health care field there is a need for a similar institution to stimulate open debate and rational learning processes by harnessing and coordinating existing and potential resources, and acting as a clearing house for the gathering and dissemination of information (McLachlan, 1990). Such a body should have a capacity to proffer advice on health policies with a fresh perspective and equally provide an independent evaluation of the impact of those policies. It would also provide a measure of public participation as public values are tightened and cemented during the processes of analysis and comment.

However, the establishment of an Institute of Health or other similar organization is by itself no guarantee of open debate and genuine accountability without supplements to Parliamentary procedures such as freedom of information and what is known as 'sunshine' legislation to open up and place on record major issues of health policy planning. The object of accountability is to ensure openness at all stages of the decisional process, thus 'policy making must be observed by arc light and not by lightning' (Harden and Lewis, 1986, pp. 243, 303). In the USA the 1977 Government in the Sunshine Act applies to all agencies of the executive branch of federal government and their subcommittees and advisory bodies. The Act provides that every part of every meeting shall be open to the public unless the subject matter is statutorily exempted. There are also requirements for records to be kept of closed meetings, procedures for public access to those records and rules for judicial review of any violation of the provisions of the Act.

In the UK the Public Bodies (Admissions to Meetings Act) 1960 requires full Regional and District Health Authority meetings to be held in public. Notice of the time and place of meetings must be posted at the offices of the health authority at least three clear days before the meeting, and the press (but not the general public) must be supplied with a copy of the agenda and any further particulars necessary to indicate the nature of any item, on request. However, a health authority may exclude the public, by resolution, whenever publicity would be prejudicial to the public interest by reason of the confidential nature of the business to be transacted or for other special reasons. These are very limited requirements. Much of health authority business is conducted without public scrutiny as exclusionary provisions are frequently interpreted broadly and the 1960 Act does not govern the conduct of business carried out in committees or sub-committees, which is in many cases extensive.

A survey conducted by the Community Rights Project and the Community Advisory Group concluded that secrecy was endemic in the conduct of health authority business apart from one or two limited exceptions. A significant number of health authorities failed even to comply with the minimal requirements of the Act.

To ensure resources and objectives were properly matched the NHS requires adequate investment in financial, management and information systems. A legitimate system would entail the disclosure of quality assurance data and the publication of policy, strategic management roles, and procedures for operation, so that performance can be assessed and accountability rendered transparent. With determination and forethought quality assurance and management systems, along with a more systematic use of complaints, could provide identifiable points for public access into the processes for policy formation and review. But the public also needs the support of legal processes, and in the last resort judicial intervention to advance the interests of open and accountable government and to structure and facilitate collective input and review. Quality, choice and efficiency in health care services are thus all reliant on the institutional framework for their delivery and can therefore be significantly affected by the quality of developments in law as well as the exigencies of economics and politics.

BIBLIOGRAPHY

Annas, Law, Rosenblatt and Wing (1990) *American Health Law*. Little, Brown & Co.

Association of Community Health Councils in England and Wales (ACHCEW) (1986) *Consultation and the Rights of CHCs*. Paper by Birmingham CHC. London, ACHCEW.

ACHCEW (1990) *National Health Service Complaints Procedures. A Review by ACHCEW*. London, ACHCEW.

ACHCEW (1991a) *Survey of CHC Relations with NHS Authorities*. London, ACHCEW.

ACHCEW (1991b) *From 'Citizens Charter' to 'Patients Charter'*. London, ACHCEW.

Audit Commission (1991) *How Effective is the Audit Commission?* London.

Barrett, S. and Hill, M. (1986) 'Policy, bargaining and structure in implementation theory: towards an integrated approach' in M. Goldsmith (ed.) *New Research in Central–Local Relations*. London, Gower.

Bevan, G. and Marinker, M. (1989) *Greening the White Paper: A Strategy for NHS Reform*. London, Social Market Foundation.

Birkinshaw, P. (1985) *Grievances, Remedies and the State*. London, Sweet and Maxwell.

Birkinshaw, P., Harden, I., and Lewis, N. (1990) *Government by Moonlight, the Hybrid Parts of the State*. London, Unwin Hyman.

Birkinshaw, P. and Lewis, N. (forthcoming) *Justice Against the State*. Buckingham, Open University Press.

Blumstein, J. (1984) 'Court action and agency reaction: the Hill-Burton Act as a case study', *Iowa Law Review*, 69, 1127.

Carrier, J. and Kendall, I. (1990) *Socialism and the NHS*. Avebury, Gower Publishing.

Community Rights Project and the Community Advisory Group (1990) *Health Authorities: A Closed Area of Government?* Secrets File No 17. Published jointly by the Community Rights Project and Community Advisory Group, London.

Coombs, R. and Cooper, D. (1990) *Accounting for Patients? Information Technology and the NHS White Paper; Paper No.10*. Manchester, Centre for Research on Organisations, Management and Technical Change, UMIST.

Cotterall, R. and Bercusson, B. (1988) 'Introduction: law, democracy and social justice', *Journal of Law and Society*, 15(1), 1.

Dunleavy, P. (1980) 'Professions and policy change; a model of ideological corporatism', *Public Administration Bulletin*, (36).

Dunsire, A. (1978) *Implementation in a Bureaucracy*. Oxford, Martin Robertson.

Enthoven, A. (1980) 'Health plan: the only practical solution to the soaring cost of medical care', *Vanderbilt Law Review*, 51.

Enthoven, A. (1988) 'Managed competition: an agenda for action', *Health Affairs*, Summer.

Enthoven, A. (1989) 'Words from the source: an interview with Alain Enthoven', *BMJ NHS Review*, 298, 1166.

Flynn, R. (1990) *Managed Markets: Consumers and Producers in the NHS*. Paper presented to *The British Sociology Association Conference*, April.

Galligan, D. (1982) 'Judicial review and the textbook writers', *Oxford Journal of Legal Studies*, (2), 257.

Graham, C. and Prosser, T. (eds) (1988) *Waiving the Rules: The Constitution under Thatcherism*. Milton Keynes, Open University Press.

Griffiths, R. (1983) *NHS Management Enquiry*. London, DHSS.

Griggs, E. (1990) *The Politics of Health Care Reform in Britain*. PSA Conference Paper, April.

Ham, C. (1990) *The New National Health Service*. Oxford, National Association of Health Authorities and Trusts.

Harden, I. (1992) *The Contracting State*. Buckingham, Open University Press.

Harden, I. and Lewis, N. (1986) *The Noble Lie: The British Constitution and the Rule of Law*. London, Hutchinson.

Harvey, S. (1991) 'Giving them what they want', *Health Service Journal*, 19 May.

Health Service Commissioner. *Annual Reports 1986–91*. London, HMSO.

Health Service Commissioner (1989) *House of Commons 2nd Report from the Select Committee on the Parliamentary Commissioner for Administration Session 1988/89. Report of the Health Service Commissioner for 1987/88 HC 433*. London, HMSO.

HMSO (1988) *Improving Management in Government; the Next Steps 1988*. London, Efficiency Unit, HMSO.

HMSO (1991) *Making the Most of Next Steps: The Management of Ministers' Departments and their Executive Agencies*. London, Efficiency Unit, HMSO.

Hogg, C. (1986) *The Public and the NHS*. London, ACHCEW.

Hughes, D. (1990) 'Same words different stories', *Health Services Journal*, 22 March, 432.

Hughes, D. (1991) 'The reorganisation of the National Health Service: the rhetoric and reality of the internal market', *Modern Law Review*, 54, 88.

Jacob, J. (1991) 'Lawyers go to hospital', *Public Law*, Summer, 225.

Jost, T. (1988) 'The necessary and proper role of regulation to assure the quality of health care', *Houston Law Review*, 25, 525.

Klein, R. (1974) 'Accountability in the health service', *Political Quarterly*, 42, 364.

Klein, R. (1989) *The Politics of the NHS* (2nd edn). Harlow, Longman.

Klein, R. and Hall, P. (1974) *Caring for Quality in the Caring Services: Options for Future Policy*. Bedford Square Press.

Klein, R. and Lewis, P. (1976) *The Politics of Consumer Representation. A Study of Community Health Councils*, London, Centre for Studies in Social Policy.

Lewis, N. (1981) 'Towards a sociology of lawyering in public administration', *Northen Ireland Quarterly*, 32, 89.

Llewellyn, K. (1940) 'The normative, the legal and the law jobs', *Yale Law Journal*, 49, 1355.

Longley, D. (1990) 'Diagnostic dilemmas: Accountability in the NHS', *Public Law*, Winter.

Longley, D. (1992) *Complaints Procedures and the Reform of the NHS*. Unpublished report on hospital and general practitioner complaints during the period of the NHS re-organization for the ESRC and British Academy.

McClure, W. (1988) 'Competition and the pursuit of quality: a conversation with Walter McClure', *Health Affairs*, 7, 79–90.

McLachlan, G. (1990) *What Price Quality: The NHS in Review*. London, Nuffield Provincial Hospital Trust.

McSweeney, B. (1988) 'Accounting for the audit commission', *Political Quarterly*, 59, 28.

Maynard, A. (1987) 'Markets and health care' in A. Williams (ed.) *Health and Economics*. London, Macmillan, pp. 139-165.

Metcalfe, L. and Richards, S. (1987) *Improving Public Management*. London, Sage.

Moore, W. (1991) 'Clean sweep needed to put house in order', *Health Service Journal*, 7 March, 14.

Moran, M. (1991) *The Health Care State in Europe: Convergence or Divergence*. Paper presented to *1991 PSA Conference*.

Nichol, D. (1989) 'Strong hand with a lighter touch', *Health Service Journal*, June, 660.

Packwood, T., Keen, J. and Buxton, M. (1991) *Hospitals in Transition: The Resource Management Experiment*. Milton Keynes, Open University Press.

Parkin, A. (1985) 'Public law and the provision of health care', *Urban Law and Policy*, 101.

Peters, B. (1978) *The Politics of Bureaucracy*. New York, Longman.

Pollitt, C. (1986) 'Beyond the managerial model: the case for broadening performance assessment in government and public services', *Financial Accountability and Management*, 2(3), 155.

Pollitt, C. (1988) *Measuring Performance of Public Services: A Consumer Perspective*. London, Leverhulme Discussion Paper.

Prosser, T. (1982) 'Towards a critical public law', *Journal of Law and Society*, 9, 1.

Prosser, T. (1986) *Nationalised Industries and Political Control: Legal, Constitutional and Political Issues*. Oxford, Blackwell.

Ranson, S. and Stewart, J. (1989) 'Citizenship and government: the challenge for management in the public domain', *Political Studies*, xxxvii, 5.

Rosenblatt, R. (1978) 'Health care reform and adminstrative law: a structural approach', *Yale Law Journal*, 88(2), 243.

Rosenblatt, R. (1981) 'Health care, markets and democratic values', *Vanderbilt Law Review*, 34(4), 1067.

Rosenblum, V. (1974) 'Handling citizen initiated complaints: an introductory study of federal agency procedures and practices', *Administrative Law Review*, 26, 1.

Seneviratne, M. (1991) 'Local Government Complaints Procedures'. Unpublished PhD thesis, University of Sheffield.

Sheaff, R. (1990) *Marketing for Health Services*. Milton Keynes, Open University Press.

Sheldon, T. (1991) 'Oiling the parts for a friendlier future', *Health Service Journal*, 11 April, 10.

Small, N. (1989) *Politics and Planning in the National Health Service*, Milton Keynes, Open University Press.

Social Services Committee (1989) *Eighth Report. Resourcing the National Health Service: The Government's Plans for the Future of the National Health Service*, HC 214 III. London, HMSO.

Stewart, J. and Clarke, M. (1987) 'The public service orientation: issues and dilemmas', *Public Administration*, 65(2), 161.

Stewart, R. (1981) 'Regulation, innovation and administrative law: a conceptual framework', *California Law Review*, 69, 1256.

Stowe, K. (1988) *On Caring for the National Health*. London, Nuffield Provincial Hospital Trust.

Strong, P. and Robinson, J. (1990) *The NHS – Under New Management*. Milton Keynes, Open University Press.

Thynne, I. and Goldring, J. (1987) *Accountability and Control: Government Officials and the Exercise of Power*. Australia, Lawbook Company.

Williams, A. (ed.) (1987) *Health and Economics*. London, Macmillan.

Wood, B. (1988) 'Privatisation, local government and the health services' in C. Graham and T. Prosser (eds) *Waiving the Rules: The Constitution Under Thatcherism*. Milton Keynes, Open University Press.

Working for Patients; the Health Service in the 1990s (1989) Cmnd 555. London, HMSO. Also:

Working Paper 1 *Self-Governing Hospitals*.
Working Paper 2 *Funding and Contracts for Hospital Services*.
Working Paper 3 *Practice Budgets for General Medical Practitioners*.
Working Paper 4 *Indicative Prescribing Budgets*.
Working Paper 6 *Medical Audit*.
Working Paper 7 *NHS Consultants; Appointments, Contracts and Distinction Awards*.
Working Paper 8 *Implications for Family Practioner Committees*.
Working Paper 9 *Self-Governing Hospitals: An Initial Guide*.
Working Paper 11 *Framework for Information Systems*.
Developing Districts; 1990 EL(90)86.
NHS Trusts; A Working Guide, 1990.
Contracts for Health Services; Operational Principles, 1990.

INDEX